Polypharmacy

Editor

MARY ANN E. ZAGARIA

CLINICS IN
GERIATRIC MEDICINE

www.geriatric.theclinics.com

May 2017 • Volume 33 • Number 2

ELSEVIER

1600 John F. Kennedy Boulevard • Suite 1800 • Philadelphia, Pennsylvania, 19103-2899

http://www.theclinics.com

CLINICS IN GERIATRIC MEDICINE Volume 33, Number 2
May 2017 ISSN 0749–0690, ISBN-13: 978-0-323-52840-5

Editor: Jessica McCool
Developmental Editor: Colleen Dietzler

Clinics in Geriatric Medicine (ISSN 0749-0690) is published quarterly by Elsevier Inc., 360 Park Avenue South, New York, NY 10010-1710. Months of issue are February, May, August, and November. Business and Editorial Offices: 1600 John F. Kennedy Blvd., Suite 1800, Philadelphia, PA 191023-2899. Periodicals postage paid at New York, NY, and additional mailing offices. Subscription prices are $273.00 per year (US individuals), $590.00 per year (US institutions), $100.00 per year (US student/resident), $381.00 per year (Canadian individuals), $748.00 per year (Canadian institutions), $195.00 per year (Canadian student/resident), $402.00 per year (international individuals), $748.00 per year (international institutions), and $195.00 per year (international student/resident). Foreign air speed delivery is included in all *Clinics* subscription prices. All prices are subject to change without notice. POSTMASTER: Send address changes to *Clinics in Geriatric Medicine,* Elsevier Health Sciences Division, Subscription Customer Service, 3251 Riverport Lane, Maryland Heights, MO 63043. **Telephone: 1-800-654-2452 (U.S. and Canada); 314-447-8871 (outside U.S. and Canada). Fax: 314-447-8029. E-mail:** journalscustomerservice-usa@elsevier.com **(for print support) or** journalsonlinesupport-usa@elsevier.com **(for online support).**

Reprints. For copies of 100 or more, of articles in this publication, please contact the Commercial Reprints Department, Elsevier Inc., 360 Park Avenue South, New York, New York 10010-1710. Tel.: 212-633-3874; Fax: 212-633-3820, E-mail: reprints@elsevier.com.

Clinics in Geriatric Medicine is covered in *MEDLINE/PubMed (Index Medicus), EMBASE/Excerpta Medica, Current Contents/Clinical Medicine (CC/CM),* and the *Cumulative Index to Nursing & Allied Health Literature.*

Contributors

EDITOR

MARY ANN E. ZAGARIA, PharmD, MS, BCGP
Clinical Consultant Pharmacist in Geriatrics and President, MZ Associates Inc, Hallowell, Maine

AUTHORS

KEVIN T. BAIN, PharmD, MPH
Vice President, Medication Risk Mitigation, Tabula Rasa HealthCare, Inc, Moorestown, New Jersey; Adjunct Faculty, Department of Pharmacy, University of the Sciences, Philadelphia College of Pharmacy, Philadelphia, Pennsylvania

NICOLE J. BRANDT, PharmD, MBA, CGP, BCGP, FASCP
Professor, Geriatric Pharmacotherapy, Department of Pharmacy Practice and Science, Executive Director, Peter Lamy Center Drug Therapy and Aging, University of Maryland School of Pharmacy, Baltimore, Maryland

ANTHONY BUONANNO, MD, MBA
Vice Chairman, Emergency and Hospital Medicine, Clinical Assistant Professor, University of South Florida Morsani College of Medicine, Medical Director of Nutrition Support Team, Lehigh Valley Health Network, Allentown, Pennsylvania

ZHE CHEN, MD
Assistant Site Leader of Hospital Medicine, Lehigh Valley Hospital Cedar Crest, Clinical Assistant Professor, University of South Florida Morsani College of Medicine, Allentown, Pennsylvania

CATHERINE E. COOKE, PharmD, BCPS, PAHM
Research Associate Professor, Department of Pharmacy Practice and Science, University of Maryland School of Pharmacy, Baltimore, Maryland

JOHN W. DEVLIN, PharmD, FCCM, FCCP
Division of Pulmonary, Critical Care and Sleep Medicine, Tufts Medical Center, School of Pharmacy, Northeastern University, Boston, Massachusetts

MICHELLE A. FRITSCH, PharmD
Founder and President, Meds MASH, LLC, Monkton, Maryland

ERIK GARPESTAD, MD, FACP, FCCM, FCCP
Division of Pulmonary, Critical Care, and Sleep Medicine, Tufts Medical Center, Boston, Massachusetts

LINDA G. GOOEN, PharmD, MS
Board Certified Geriatric Pharmacist, Fellow American Society of Consultant Pharmacists, Gooen Consulting, LLC, Basking Ridge, New Jersey; Adjunct Assistant Clinical Professor, Pharmacy Practice and Administration, Ernest P. Mario School of Pharmacy, Rutgers University, New Brunswick, New Jersey

HOLLY M. HOLMES, MD, MS
Division of Geriatric and Palliative Medicine, University of Texas Health McGovern Medical School, Houston, Texas

TAHA KHAN, PharmD, RPh
The Access Group, Berkeley Heights, New Jersey

CALVIN H. KNOWLTON, BPharm, MDiv, PhD
CEO, Tabula Rasa HealthCare, Inc, Moorestown, New Jersey

HEDVA BARENHOLTZ LEVY, PharmD, BCPS, BCGP
Director, HbL PharmaConsulting, St Louis, Missouri

PENNY S. SHELTON, PharmD
Executive Director, North Carolina Association of Pharmacists, Durham, North Carolina

RICHARD G. STEFANACCI, DO, MGH, MBA, AGSF, CMD
The Access Group, Berkeley Heights, New Jersey; Thomas Jefferson University, College of Population Health, Philadelphia, Pennsylvania

ADAM TODD, PhD, MPharm
Division of Pharmacy, School of Medicine, Pharmacy and Health, Durham University, Stockton-on-Tees, United Kingdom

JACQUES TURGEON, BPharm, PhD
Chief Scientific Officer, Tabula Rasa HealthCare, Inc, Moorestown, New Jersey; Adjunct Professor, Department of Systems Pharmacology and Translational Therapeutics, University of Pennsylvania, Philadelphia, Pennsylvania; Adjunct Professor, Department of Pharmaceutics, College of Pharmacy, University of Florida, Gainesville, Florida; Professor Emeritus, Universitè de Montréal, Montreal, Quebec, Canada

Contents

Centers for Medicare and Medicaid Services Support for Medication Therapy Management (Enhanced Medication Therapy Management): Testing Strategies for Improving Medication Use Among Beneficiaries Enrolled in Medicare Part D

Nicole J. Brandt and Catherine E. Cooke

In 2006, Medicare beneficiaries began receiving prescription coverage benefits through Part D of the Medicare benefit. Medicare Part D plans must provide medication therapy (MTM) services. MTM services aim to improve medication use and are targeted toward eligible beneficiaries, determined by morbidity, prescription use, and anticipated cost of prescription use. Now, 10 years after the start of Medicare Part D, several changes have been made to the program's design. This article focuses on changes related to MTM and the impact that these changes have and will continue to have on Medicare beneficiaries and medication use.

The Role of Patient Preferences in Deprescribing

Holly M. Holmes and Adam Todd

Polypharmacy and the use of inappropriate medications has become an increasing problem globally. Deprescribing has gained attention as a means to rationalize medication use. Deprescribing interventions have been shown to be generally feasible and safe; in the few studies in which patient preferences are assessed, such interventions also seem to be acceptable to patients. Qualitative studies suggest that patients are interested in reducing medications, may need education about their medications to facilitate deprescribing, and highly value communication with their providers around deprescribing. This article focuses on patient preferences for deprescribing and highlights practical recommendations to overcome barriers to deprescribing.

Polypharmacy Reduction Strategies: Tips on Incorporating American Geriatrics Society Beers and Screening Tool of Older People's Prescriptions Criteria

Hedva Barenholtz Levy

There is no single definition of polypharmacy. Use of 5 or more medications commonly is used. An alternative, quantitative definition, such as use of more medications than clinically indicated or use of unnecessary or harmful prescribing, has been proposed. Protocols or algorithms to improve polypharmacy and prescribing in older adults have been developed. The American Geriatrics Society (AGS) Beers Criteria and Screening Tool of Older People's Prescriptions (STOPP) explicit criteria reflect elements that are common across protocols and algorithms. Concepts in AGS Beers and STOPP can be incorporated into polypharmacy reduction strategies to improve outcomes of care for older adults.

CLINICS IN GERIATRIC MEDICINE

ISSUE OF RELATED INTEREST

Clinics in Geriatric Medicine, May 2012 (Vol. 28, No. 2)
Polypharmacy
Holly M. Holmes, *Editor*
http://www.geriatric.theclinics.com

THE CLINICS ARE AVAILABLE ONLINE!
Access your subscription at:
www.theclinics.com

Preface

Inroads into Polypharmacy: Moving Forward with Tools, Deprescribing, and Philosophical Reflection

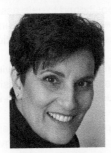

Mary Ann E. Zagaria, PharmD, MS, BCGP
Editor

Clinicians who care for older adults and strive to improve quality of care wrestle with the ongoing burden of polypharmacy and the balance between underprescribing and overprescribing. In addition, the ability for patients to purchase medications online and through channels that do not carefully monitor quality or quantity of drugs is likely to continue to increase and complicate polypharmacy-related problems.

This special issue of *Clinics in Geriatric Medicine* has been developed to address polypharmacy from a comprehensive yet practical approach. It provides updated evidence, tools, and insight from authors with expertise in geriatric medicine and pharmacy, and commitment to and compassion for, the geriatric individuals they serve. The variety of practice settings covered in this issue, from primary care to critical care, from assisted living and long-term care, and from an academic-based clinic perspective to a managed care perspective, underscores the growing need for geriatrics integration throughout the health care system and continuum of care. It is truly a manual of sorts for making inroads into polypharmacy.

Brandt and Cooke focus on changes to Medication Therapy Management and the impact they will have on Medicare beneficiaries and medication utilization. They discuss the evolution of the Medicare Part D Medication Therapy Management overseen by Centers for Medicare and Medicaid Services and the implications on addressing polypharmacy.

Holmes and Todd focus on patient preferences for deprescribing and patient-centered care in guiding deprescribing interventions. They address the process of deprescribing and highlight practical recommendations to overcome barriers to the process.

Clin Geriatr Med 33 (2017) ix–x
http://dx.doi.org/10.1016/j.cger.2017.02.001
0749-0690/17/© 2017 Published by Elsevier Inc.

While highlighting trends in medication use among older adults, Levy discusses systematic approaches to address polypharmacy and guides clinicians in applying the American Geriatrics Society (AGS) Beers 2015 and Screening Tool of Older People's Prescriptions (STOPP) version 2 criteria as a framework for evaluating polypharmacy regimens and reducing polypharmacy.

Garpestad and Devlin hone in on recognition and prevention of polypharmacy and delirium in critically ill older adults. They address specific pharmacologic ICU delirium treatment interventions and strategies on how to recognize and reduce medication-associated delirium.

Shelton and Fritsch discuss pharmacists as members of the interprofessional health care team and discuss how these clinicians are uniquely positioned to help assess and address falls risk. They discuss a six-step, comprehensive falls assessment, including falls-associated drugs and medical conditions, and describe implementation concepts based on the pharmacy practice setting.

In addressing medication reconciliation in long-term care and in assisted living facilities, Gooen lays out the opportunity to minimize risks associated with transitions of care, discusses electronic health care records, and includes case studies and common barriers to the medication reconciliation process.

Key opportunities for managed care to manage polypharmacy are presented by Stefanacci and Khan. Discussing another value-based care model, which involves a health care delivery concept that provides an alternate understanding of how primary care is organized and delivered, the authors indicate how it will exist in most care settings rather than being isolated in only managed care organizations or HMOs.

Bain and colleagues show how pharmacists, through their training in pharmacodynamics, pharmacokinetics, and medication management, are ideally qualified to mitigate medication risk through traditional and enhanced strategies, including innovative drug interaction tools and pharmacogenomics, and the integration of the same into clinical practice.

Last, a special feature of this issue includes up close and personal accounts from two physicians, Buonanno and Chen, sharing their candid experiences with polypharmacy, including one as a caregiver for a family member, in the true spirit of philosophical reflection to raise awareness and improve care.

The contributions of these extraordinary authors brought together for this issue addressing polypharmacy aim to provide strategies, practical measures, and insight to clinicians and those who educate, develop public policy, and guide public health campaigns. In addition, we hope to stimulate thought, encourage conversation, and inspire the next generation of clinicians charged with serving our vulnerable elders, active or frail, of today and tomorrow.

Mary Ann E. Zagaria, PharmD, MS, BCGP
PO Box 327
Hallowell, ME 04347, USA

E-mail address:
mzagaria@mzassociatesinc.com

Centers for Medicare and Medicaid Services Support for Medication Therapy Management (Enhanced Medication Therapy Management)

Testing Strategies for Improving Medication Use Among Beneficiaries Enrolled in Medicare Part D

Nicole J. Brandt, PharmD, MBA, CGP, BCGP[a],*,
Catherine E. Cooke, PharmD, BCPS, PAHM[b]

KEYWORDS

- Medication therapy management ● Part D prescription drug benefit
- Centers for Medicare and Medicaid Services ● Drug therapy problems

KEY POINTS

- With the implementation of Medicare Part D prescription drug coverage, eligible Medicare beneficiaries now have access to MTM services. The requirements for MTM have evolved since its inception affording providers the opportunity to improve care delivery.
- As MTM providers, pharmacists are integral to the success of ensuring appropriate medication use throughout the care continuum for older adults.
- The ongoing "enhanced" MTM initiative will inform the industry on best practices for MTM and help ideally to create future standards.

Older adults in the United States use a disproportionate amount of medications. Because the number of medications has been shown to be a strong predictor for medication-related problems, it is no surprise that older adults are at greater risk.[1] This problem spans beyond the health and well-being of the elderly by also raising

Disclosure Statement: Drs N.J. Brandt and C.E. Cooke have served as clinical consultants on grants with Econometrica, Inc and Impaq International, LLC with work focused on medication therapy management for Medicare beneficiaries.
[a] Geriatric Pharmacotherapy, Department of Pharmacy Practice and Science, Peter Lamy Center Drug Therapy and Aging, University of Maryland School of Pharmacy, 20 North Pine Street N529, Baltimore, MD 21201, USA; [b] Department of Pharmacy Practice and Science, University of Maryland School of Pharmacy, 20 North Pine Street, Baltimore, MD 21201, USA
* Corresponding author.
E-mail address: nbrandt@rx.umaryland.edu

the financial burden of health care. According to a recent study, the misuse of medications contributes to $500 billion in international health care spending and more work needs to be done to focus on older adults.[2] In America, medication-related problems in the older adult population are associated with an annual expense of $8 billion.[3] With the US aged population growing at a faster rate than ever before, the need to ensure safe medication management for older adults presents an urgent need in the health care community. This article discusses the evolution of the Medicare Part D medication therapy management (MTM) program overseen by the Centers for Medicare and Medicaid Services (CMS) and the implications on addressing polypharmacy.

BACKGROUND

"Medication therapy management is a service or group of services that optimizes therapeutic outcomes for individual patients. MTM services include medication therapy reviews, pharmacotherapy consults, anticoagulation management, immunizations, health and wellness programs and many other clinical services. Pharmacists provide MTM to help patients get the best benefits from their medications by actively managing drug therapy and by identifying, preventing and resolving medication-related problems."[4] In 2006, the Medicare Part D prescription drug benefit program began through insurance companies as a voluntary program. It was required that every Part D plan offer an MTM program to improve the quality of prescribing. The requirements for MTM programs: under 423.153(d), a Part D sponsor must have established an MTM program that ensures optimum therapeutic outcomes for targeted beneficiaries through improved medication use, reduces the risk of adverse events, is developed with licensed and practicing pharmacists and physicians, describes the resources and time required to implement the program, establishes the fees for MTM providers, and may be furnished by pharmacists or other qualified providers.

The initial CMS regulations established a general framework for providing MTM services, allowing Medicare Part D plan sponsors flexibility to promote best practices. Annually, Part D sponsors must submit MTM program descriptions for CMS to review and approve. After analyzing common practices, CMS significantly enhanced the requirements for MTM programs starting in 2010. There were more robust requirements for MTM programs including reporting and documenting that have evolved since 2006. **Fig. 1** displays the key changes in the requirements, discussed in the upcoming sections.

MEDICATION THERAPY MANAGEMENT PROGRAM TARGETING REQUIREMENTS

In general, each Medicare Part D program must enroll targeted beneficiaries using an opt-out method when they meet the eligibility criteria. Since the start of the MTM program in 2006, the main components of eligibility have remained, and include the number of disease states, the number of medications, and a cost threshold. For 2017, the following sections describe the minimum eligibility requirements as put forth by CMS, but plans have the choice to be less restrictive with their criteria.[5]

Multiple Chronic Conditions

Beneficiaries must have multiple chronic diseases, with three chronic diseases being the maximum number a Part D plan sponsor may require for targeted enrollment. Of note, sponsors may set this minimum threshold at two or three. Additionally, Part D sponsors may target beneficiaries with any chronic diseases or target beneficiaries

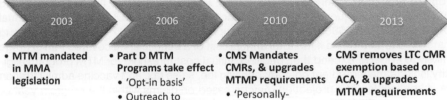

| 2003 | 2006 | 2010 | 2013 |

- MTM mandated in MMA legislation

- Part D MTM Programs take effect
  - 'Opt-in basis'
  - Outreach to beneficiaries and providers (through mail, call centers and face-to-face meetings)

- CMS Mandates CMRs, & upgrades MTMP requirements
  - 'Personally-delivered' CMR
  - 'Opt-out' enrollment
  - Beginnings of interactive consultations

- CMS removes LTC CMR exemption based on ACA, & upgrades MTMP requirements
  - Standard formats
  - Targeting criterias updated
  - Creation of a special criteria for cognitively impaired
  - LTC beneficiaries and CMS

Fig. 1. Key changes in MTM requirements. ACA, Affordable Care Act; CMR, comprehensive medication review; LTC, long-term care; MMA, Medicare Modernization Act; MTMP, medication therapy management programs.

with specific chronic diseases. However, if sponsors choose to target beneficiaries with specific chronic diseases, they should include conditions from at least five of the nine core chronic conditions in **Box 1**.

Multiple Covered Part D Drugs

Based on plan design alone, Medicare beneficiaries that are enrolled in the program have "polypharmacy." They are taking multiple Part D drugs, with eight Part D drugs being the maximum number of drugs a Part D plan sponsor may require as the minimum number of Part D drugs that a beneficiary must be taking for targeted enrollment.

Anticipated Part D Drug Costs

Furthermore, targeted enrollees are likely to incur annual costs for covered Part D drugs greater than or equal to the specified MTM cost threshold. In 2006, the MTM

Box 1
CMS-defined core chronic conditions

- Alzheimer's disease
- Chronic heart failure
- Diabetes
- Dyslipidemia
- End-stage renal disease
- Hypertension
- Respiratory disease (eg, asthma, chronic obstructive pulmonary disease, or chronic lung disorders)
- Bone disease–arthritis (eg, osteoporosis, osteoarthritis, or rheumatoid arthritis)
- Mental health (eg, depression, schizophrenia, bipolar disorder, or chronic/disabling mental health conditions)

program annual cost threshold was $4000. However, in 2009, this was lowered to $3000, with subsequent small annual increases since then.[6] In 2016, the annual cost threshold was $3507, whereas the updated one for 2017 is $3919.[4] The drug costs used to determine if the total annual cost of a beneficiary's covered Part D drugs is likely to equal or exceed the specified annual cost threshold for MTM program eligibility include the ingredient cost, dispensing fee, sales tax, and vaccine administration fee, if applicable. This projection may be based on claims within the program year or based on historical claims from the previous year.

Part D plan sponsors are encouraged to optimize their MTM programs, including their targeting criteria, to offer MTM to beneficiaries who will benefit the most from these services.[7] Beneficiaries are considered enrolled unless they decline or permanently opt out of the MTM program for the current or future years. Of note, plan sponsors are expected to use more than one approach when possible to reach all eligible beneficiaries and target them at least quarterly during each year. Furthermore, to improve continuity of care, the plans are expected to perform an analysis at the end of the year to identify current MTM program participants to prevent interruption of MTM interventions.

Ongoing attention is being given to the targeting requirements because of the complexity of the design and the lack of clarity on understanding who is eligible for MTM services, and when they are eligible for these services. This may be in part caused by the design of the MTM program being an administrative cost to plans and depending on their incentives may not be a priority. However, changes to quality metrics, such as the star rating system which includes a measure of the completion rate of comprehensive medications reviews (CMRs), may better align incentives.

MEDICATION THERAPY MANAGEMENT PROGRAM DOCUMENTATION AFTER A COMPREHENSIVE MEDICATION REVIEW: THE STANDARDIZED FORMAT

With respect to documentation, there were changes within the Patient Protection and Affordable Care Act of 2010 that directed CMS, in consultation with relevant stakeholders, to develop a formal template, referred to as the Standardized Format (SF), to document the medication-related action plan and the summary of the CMR. The CMR is an interactive session with the beneficiary and qualified MTM provider where medications are reviewed, drug therapy problems (DTPs) are identified, and a plan for resolution is developed. The CMR must be delivered person-to-person or using tele-health technologies by a licensed pharmacist or other qualified provider, with a written medication review and action plan and input from the prescriber as necessary and practical. On January 1, 2013, all patients receiving a CMR were required to receive a written summary of the encounter using the MTM SF.

The SF includes three components (cover letter, medication action plan, and personal medication list), and must be provided to the patient within 14 days. The new requirement for the SF after a CMR advanced consistency in the service by providing a template of content to be expected from a CMR. However, barriers to integrate the SF into existing electronic medical records remain. The SF focuses on the needs of the beneficiary, which may not be interoperable with existing electronic medical documentation because of variations in terminology. Several organizations, such as the Pharmacy HIT Collaborative, are working to create processes to integrate information from the SF into current medical practice.[8] Further work is necessary to develop a consensus about how best to facilitate these processes to improve patient outcomes related to medication use and safety.

MEDICATION THERAPY MANAGEMENT WITHIN THE LONG-TERM CARE SETTING: COMPREHENSIVE MEDICATION REVIEW AND BENEFICIARIES

With respect to implementation across various practice settings, effective January 1, 2013, Medicare Modernization Act (MMA) Sec. 1860D 4(c) (2) (A) (ii) – Medicare Part D Required MTM for targeted beneficiaries noted that implementing regulations at 423.154(d) (1) (vii) (B)[6]:

- The Affordable Care Act as amended in section 10,328 does not provide a basis for creating an exception to the requirement to offer a CMR based on the setting of care.
- Targeted beneficiaries in other health care settings are not excluded from the Part D MTM requirements, and must be offered MTM services.

Pharmacists who work in long-term care (LTC) settings, such as nursing homes, are already providing clinical services. **Table 1** differentiates the types of medication-related services that are currently performed in LTC facilities: CMR, monthly Drug Regimen Review, and Targeted Medication Review.[9,10]

CMS, within the April 2012 ruling, states: "We agree that the LTC consultant pharmacists would be a valuable resource for the delivery of CMRs to targeted beneficiaries in LTC settings...we encourage plan sponsors to consider making arrangements that include the LTC consultant pharmacist in conducting Part D MTM services for targeted beneficiaries in LTC."[11] Despite this suggestion it is unclear how Medicare Part D plans are operationalizing CMRs for their beneficiaries in LTC. Coordination of care initiatives among health care professionals is known to improve the quality of patient care.

This is evidenced by a recent partnership between a health plan and an LTC pharmacy provider whereby consultant pharmacists provided CMRs for their LTC beneficiaries using the 2013 CMS SF.[12] The LTC pharmacy provider's proprietary consultant

Table 1
Differentiating medication-related services in LTC

CMR[9]	DRR[10]	TMR[9]
• Annual, comprehensive	• Monthly (once every 30 d)	• Quarterly
• Only for targeted beneficiaries	• Conducted with every resident	• Specific or potential medication and/or medication-related problems
• Recommendations provided to resident	• Recommendations provided to nursing staff and prescriber	
• Language understandable for beneficiary	• Summary is written in professional language	
• Interactive, person-to-person or telehealth medication review	• Review of medications over 10-min intervals	
• Expected to take 45–60 min		

Abbreviations: DRR, drug regimen review; TMR, targeted medication review.

Data from Department of Health and Human Services. Centers for Medicare & Medicaid Services. Correction - CY 2017 Medication Therapy Management Program Guidance and Submission Instructions. Available at: https://www.cms.gov/Medicare/Prescription-Drug-Coverage/PrescriptionDrugCov Contra/Downloads/Memo-Contract-Year-2017-Medication-Therapy-Management-MTM-Program-Submission-v-040816.pdf. Accessed August 4, 2016; and CMS Manual System. Department of Health & Human Services (DHHS). Pub. 100-07 State Operations. Provider Certification. Centers for Medicare & Medicaid Services (CMS). pp508. Available at: https://www.cms.gov/Regulations-and-Guidance/Guidance/Transmittals/downloads/R22SOMA.pdf. Accessed August 4, 2016.

pharmacist software was programmed to produce a cover letter, medication action plan, and personal medication list per CMS specifications; their consultant pharmacists were trained to perform CMRs and the interactive interviews using this system. MTM-eligible Medicare Part D beneficiaries were identified by the health plan as residing in a skilled nursing facility (SNF) serviced by the LTC pharmacy provider; they were then provided a CMR and written summary in CMS SF by consultant pharmacists. Residents with cognitive impairment were identified using three data elements in the Minimum Data Set, including the Brief Interview for Mental Status Summary Score as interpreted by surveyors of LTC facilities in Appendix PP of the Guide for Surveyors of Long-term Care Facilities.

Through the end of November 2013, there were 1538 of 2323 beneficiaries identified as residing in nursing facilities serviced by the consultant pharmacists working for the LTC pharmacy provider. Only 38 (2.4%) residents refused CMR and 1411 of 1500 (94%) were completed successfully. There were 622 (44%) residents with cognitive impairment per Minimum Data Set assessments; CMRs were conducted with someone other than the beneficiary in those instances. However, the CMR was conducted with the beneficiary in 56% of cases. More than 2200 DTP recommendations were made to prescribers as a result of these MTM services, which led to 610 DTP resolutions, including reductions in polypharmacy, high-risk medications, and antipsychotic use and dosage. Consultant pharmacists viewed the CMR process as a rewarding, yet challenging experience at times, that favorably impacted resident care and medication understanding, and was well-received by residents and other CMR recipients.[12]

INCREASING BENEFICIARY AWARENESS OF MEDICATION THERAPY MANAGEMENT

CMS has undertaken several initiatives to improve beneficiary awareness of the value of MTM services. Over the years there has been a multifaceted education approach through

- Expanded information about MTM in the Medicare and You Handbook starting in 2013
- Easier access to plan-specific MTM information within Medicare Plan Finder
- Consistent information about MTM services on Part D plan Web sites
- CMS encouraged Medicare Part D plan outreach to promote beneficiary participation in MTM services

Pharmacists continue to promote the value added of MTM and barriers that need to be overcome to help patients (beneficiaries) access this service.[13]

MEDICATION THERAPY MANAGEMENT PROGRAMS IMPACTED BY CENTERS FOR MEDICARE AND MEDICAID SERVICES STAR MEASURE RATINGS

To provide beneficiaries with consumer-driven information about the available Part D plans, CMS began publishing a rating system, often referred to as "star ratings." This system uses a range of stars (from one to five stars) to denote how the plan is doing with a specific measure, and overall. Five stars equates to excellent performance, whereas one star means poor performance. Plans were slow to pay attention to star ratings. However, they have grown in importance. With the passage of the Affordable Care Act in 2010, financial incentives in the form of bonus payments for health plans (ie, Medicare Advantage plans) began to be tied, in certain circumstances, to star ratings.

There are several star rating measures that relate to medication use. Although these measures are important on their own, they are not equally weighted toward the overall, or summary, score for the plan. Some measures have a higher weight and therefore earn greater attention by the health plan, because they have a greater impact on overall score. For example, there is a greater weight placed on medication adherence (eg, adherence to noninsulin diabetes medications, statins, and renin angiotensin system antagonists, such as angiotensin-converting enzyme inhibitors, angiotensin receptor blockers, and aliskiren), than for the completion rates for the annual CMR for patients enrolled in the MTM program. CMS assigns star ratings based on the plan achieving a certain percentage for each measure. For example, the cut points to earn stars for the plan's CMR completion rate are presented in **Table 2** for two different types of Part D plans, prescription drug plans (PDPs) and Medicare Advantage Prescription Drug plans. The role of MTM is further supported within these Part D measures because MTM programs have been shown to improve the measures that affect star ratings. In Connecticut, a study found that of the 971 DTPs found in 88 beneficiaries, 26.2% were related to nonadherence, and 22.7% of them were lacking a necessary therapy.[14] Providing MTM to these patients improved these measures that directly affect star ratings. In addition, many MTM programs began targeting high-risk medications to address the Part D measure, appropriate use of high-risk medications in patients 65 years and older. Although these measures are highlights of medication-related Part D measures for 2016, the measures change. Some measures are retired, some are modified, and new measures are created.

THE FUTURE OF MEDICATION THERAPY MANAGEMENT: THE "ENHANCED" MEDICATION THERAPY MANAGEMENT MODEL

The CMS Innovation Center (CMMI) was established by the ACA to test payment and service delivery models to determine their effect on expenditures and quality of care for existing programs. At the end of 2016, CMMI unveiled the long-awaited "enhanced" MTM model pilot (http://innovation.cms.gov/initiatives/enhancedmtm/index.html), which is a 5-year pilot to ramp up incentives to MTM for stand-alone PDPs in five test regions. The selected five regions and corresponding states are Region 7 (Virginia), Region 11 (Florida), Region 21 (Louisiana), Region 25 (Iowa, Minnesota, Montana, Nebraska, North Dakota, South Dakota, Wyoming), and Region 28 (Arizona).

Unlike Medicare Advantage plans that are responsible for medical and prescription costs, stand-alone PDPs are responsible for only the prescription costs. PDPs have not had easy access to medical data for their beneficiaries and often cannot see, nor financially benefit from, higher cost therapies that offset or lower medical

Table 2 Star rating cutoffs for MTM-eligible program enrollees who received a CMR during the reporting period		
Star Rating	Prescription Drug Plan, %	Medicare Advantage Plans, %
5 Stars	>36.7	>76.0
4 Stars	>27.2 to <36.7	>48.6 to <76.0
3 Stars	>16.6 to <27.2	>36.2 to <48.6
2 Stars	>8.5 to <16.6	>13.6 to <36.2
1 Star	<8.5	<13.6

From Five Star Quality Rating System. Available at: https://www.cms.gov/medicare/provider-enrollment-and-certification/certificationandcomplianc/fsqrs.html. Accessed June 28, 2016.

expenditures. To align incentives, the enhanced MTM model will provide medical data and pay PDPs extra money to provide MTM that is intended to achieve the CMS triple aim. Plan sponsors will have the flexibility to offer different levels and types of MTM services and cost-sharing assistance to beneficiaries, instead of providing the same level to all targeted individuals. Plan sponsors will not be required to limit interventions to predefined beneficiary categories, but will be required to submit written plans for their proposed protocols outlining how they will target beneficiaries. A plan sponsor may exit the model after the completion of any 1 year, but no new sponsors may join after the first year. Furthermore, the plans must have a Part D summary score of three stars or higher and those plans with fewer stars may be eligible to participate but need to provide additional justification.

CMS will assess whether providing Part D sponsors with additional payment incentives (**Table 3**) and MTM regulatory flexibilities, for PDP Basic Plans, better achieves the key goals of MTM. With respect to regulatory flexibility, the PDP can vary the intensity and types of MTM services offered to enrollees based on beneficiary risk level. CMS will not specify either targeting criteria or intervention activities, preferring participating plan sponsors design, experiment with, and seek a range of strategies. CMS-standardized language and formats are not required for beneficiaries who receive the services.

CMS intends to provide participating sponsors with beneficiary Medicare Parts A and B claims data on request, which will help with optimizing the delivery of MTM. Also a uniform set of data elements, including information on specific beneficiary-level interventions and outcomes, will be collected as a condition for model test participation. CMS intends to collect encounter data including dates and provider identifiers where possible to assess sponsor performance with respect to their CMS-approved intervention plans. Additionally, the enhanced MTM will also be the "testing" area for various health information technology initiatives. Ideally, standardized approaches

Table 3
CMS financial incentives for part D sponsors

Prospective Payment	Performance Payment
• A direct payment to PDPs to support the cost of the expansion interventions; will be paid on a PMPM basis.	• $2 PMPM to plans that are successful in improving outcomes and reducing Part A/B expenditures.
• The actual cost of this PMPM payment will vary by plan and be determined by the specific interventions proposed by the plans.	• CMS is setting a minimum savings rate of 2% (net of prospective payment), to qualify for the performance payment.
• Actual PMPM prospective payment amounts will be based on the cost assumptions embedded in participating plans' approved applications spread across the entire projected plan enrollment.	• This performance-based payment will be in the form of an increase in government contribution to the plan premium.
• The approved PMPM amounts will be paid per enrollee in the plan regardless of how many of those enrollees are receiving the enhanced MTM items or services.	

Abbreviation: PMPM, per member per month.

From Centers for Medicare & Medicaid Services. Part D enhanced medication therapy management model. Available at: https://www.cms.gov/medicare/provider-enrollment-and-certification/certificationandcomplianc/fsqrs.html. Accessed August 4, 2016.

to coding and data exchange will be created that will ultimately help with looking at the quality of the MTM program.

In 2013, the Health IT Policy Committee Certification and Adoption Workgroup suggested the incorporation of an electronic health record certification program, supporting the adoption of electronic health records by pharmacists in medication management settings, creating a common platform for providers in different care settings to support smooth exchange of standard, interoperable clinical data to improve care delivery.[15] Furthermore, the Office of the National Coordinator for Health Information Technology 2014 standards require that electronic health record technology uses Systematized Nomenclature of Medicine – Clinical Terms (SNOMED CT) to denote patient clinical conditions, which is practical and ideal for practitioners during an episode of care.[16] The use of SNOMED CT codes improves communication between health care providers and care transitions through interoperability and a universal coding language, allowing more information to be available quickly and sorted easily to assist real-time decision-making.[11] Technical information and files for download are accessed at https://www.nlm.nih.gov/research/umls/Snomed/us_edition.html.

CLINICAL IMPLICATIONS FOR OLDER ADULTS

There are many implications of MTM services on the care of older adults with respect to polypharmacy and other DTPs. Resolution of these issues may result from interventions made to the patient or their health care team based on the information gathered during MTM services. DTPs can be identified and resolved by pharmacists in the community pharmacy practice setting and more integrated delivery systems.[17,18] The normal protocol for pharmacists to resolve such problems is via a recommendation to the patient directly, an offer to contact the patient's physician directly, or a recommendation that the patient follow up with their general physician. Of note, many DTPs are resolved without the direct involvement of the prescriber, because one study reported that 80% of DTPs did not require the direct involvement of a physician.[19] The most common resolutions included patient education (35.8%), elimination of a barrier to access a medication (26.8%), initiation of a new drug therapy (11.8%), and change in dose (10.5%). Resolution of DTPs that required physician involvement included initiation of a new drug therapy (32.4%), change in drug dosage (25.2%), change in drug product (14.7%), and discontinuation of a drug therapy (12.1%).

Although some studies report high rates of prescriber acceptance of recommendations, these studies are typically in more integrated systems.[13] In community pharmacy, physicians accepted 47.4% of pharmacist-recommended changes to drug therapy.[20] Physician agreement was highest with recommendations to stop or change a medication (50.3% and 50.0%, respectively) and lowest with starting a new medication (41.7%). Similar results were found in a study by Leikola and colleagues,[21] which noted that more than half of all pharmacist recommendations from CMRs were accepted by physicians and most often resulted in change of drug therapy, particularly stopping a specific drug regimen. From the various interventions in effect, one study showed that safety initiatives often have a high rate of acceptance by providers.[22] Other categories, such as medication adherence, are equally critical and can improve health and reduce costs.[23]

A study of pharmacist-provided CMR to Medicare beneficiaries in community pharmacies demonstrated improvements in medication adherence for patients taking medications for cholesterol management, gastroesophageal reflux disease, and thyroid and benign prostatic hyperplasia.[24] Several other studies support pharmacist-provided MTM by demonstrating increased medication adherence, improved health outcomes, and reduced overall medical costs.[25,26]

Additionally, innovations in health information technology present an opportunity to increase medication adherence rates, because an increasing number of consumer-facing tools are available to assist in the self-management of health conditions.[27] Identifying and resolving DTPs are of great clinical importance to care. Outcomes of resolving DTPs through provision of a CMR include an improvement in medication adherence and a decrease in the use of high-risk medications. Ultimately, to achieve desired goals of care, there needs to be ongoing collaboration among MTM providers, beneficiaries, caregivers, and the health care team to minimize DTPs and optimize patient-focused outcomes.

SUMMARY

During the last 10 years there have been valuable lessons learned about prescription coverage design and how this impacts the use of medications by Medicare beneficiaries. Studies have shown that integrated care models and data exchange are crucial to the success of MTM services. As the Medicare Part D MTM program evolves further and initiatives, such as the CMMI "enhanced" MTM, inform the industry, more changes are expected to come. National programs, such as Medicare Part D MTM, are critical to the success of combating polypharmacy in older adults and ultimately improve medication safety.

REFERENCES

1. Steinman MA, Miao Y, Boscardin WJ, et al. Prescribing quality in older veterans: a multifocal approach. J Gen Intern Med 2014;29(10):1379–86.
2. IMS Institute. IMS Institute study: $500B in global health spending can be avoided annually through more responsible use of medicines. 2012. Available at: http://www.imshealth.com/portal/site/ims/menuitem.d248e29c86589c9c30e81c033208c22a/?vgnextoid=563637d68412a310VgnVCM10000076192ca2RCRD&vgnextchannel=437879d7f269e210VgnVCM10000071812ca2RCRD&vgnextfmt=default. Accessed May 20, 2016.
3. Burton MM, Hope C, Murray MD, et al. The cost of adverse drug events in ambulatory care. AMIA Annu Symp Proc 2007;90–3.
4. What is medication therapy management? APhA MTM Central. Available at: http://www.pharmacist.com/mtm. Accessed June 30, 2016.
5. Shapiro JR. CY 2017 medication therapy management program guidance and submission instructions. [Memorandum]. Baltimore (MD): Centers for Medicare and Medicaid; 2016.
6. Federal Register: Department of Health and Human Services. Centers for Medicare & Medicaid Services, 42 CFR Parts 417, 422 and 423, Medicare Program; Changes to the Medicare Advantage and the Medicare, Prescription Drug Benefit Programs for Contract Year 2013 and Other Changes; Final Rule. Available at: https://www.gpo.gov/fdsys/pkg/FR-2012-04-12/pdf/2012-8071.pdf. Accessed August 4, 2016.
7. Wang J, Shih Y, Qin Y, et al. Trends in Medicare Part D medication. Am Health Drug Benefits 2015;8(5):247–55.
8. Cooke C, Kaiser M, Natarajan N, et al. Medicare beneficiary satisfaction with comprehensive medication review and the Standardized Format. Poster session presented at: Academy of Managed Care Pharmacy 27th Annual Meeting and Expo. Orlando (FL), October 26–29, 2015.
9. Department of Health and Human Services. Centers for Medicare & Medicaid Services. Correction - CY 2017 Medication Therapy Management Program Guidance

and Submission Instructions. Available at: https://www.cms.gov/Medicare/Prescription-Drug-Coverage/PrescriptionDrugCovContra/Downloads/Memo-Contract-Year-2017-Medication-Therapy-Management-MTM-Program-Submission-v-040816.pdf. Accessed August 4, 2016.

10. CMS Manual System. Department of Health & Human Services (DHHS). Pub. 100–07 State Operations, Provider Certification. Centers for Medicare & Medicaid Services (CMS). pp508. Available at: https://www.cms.gov/Regulations-and-Guidance/Guidance/Transmittals/downloads/R22SOMA.pdf. Accessed August 4, 2016.

11. Tudor CG. CY 2013 medication therapy management program guidance and submission instructions. [Memorandum]. Baltimore (MD): Centers for Medicare and Medicaid; 2012.

12. Brandt N, Zarowitz B. Aligning care initiatives to reduce medication adverse effects in nursing homes. J Gerontol Nurs 2015;41:8–13.

13. Gilchrist A. Pharmacy stakeholders call for strengthened MTM program. Available at: http://www.pharmacytimes.com/news/pharmacy-stakeholders-call-for-strengthened-mtm-program. Accessed June 30, 2016.

14. Smith M, Giuliano MR, Starkowski MP. In Connecticut: improving patient medication management in primary care. Health Aff (Millwood) 2011;30(4):646–54.

15. Pharmacy HIT Collaborative. The roadmap for pharmacy health information technology integration in U.S. health care. 2013. Available at: http://www.pharmacyhit.org/pdfs/11-392_RoadMapFinal_singlepages.pdf. Accessed May 20, 2016.

16. Pharmacy HIT Collaborative. Documenting comprehensive medication management in team-based models (Using SNOMED CT Codes). 2014. Available at: http://www.pharmacyhit.org/pdfs/workshop-documents/WG2-Post-2014-03.pdf. Accessed May 20, 2016.

17. Ernst ME, Doucette WR, Dedhiya SD, et al. Use of point-of-service health status assessments by community pharmacists to identify and resolve drug-related problems in patients with musculoskeletal disorders. Pharmacotherapy 2001; 21:988–97.

18. Brummel A, Lustig A, Westrich K, et al. Best practices: improving patient outcomes and costs in an ACO through comprehensive medication therapy management. J Manag Care Spec Pharm 2014;20:1152–8.

19. Ramalho de Oliveira D, Brummel AR, Miller DB. Medication therapy management: 10 years of experience in a large integrated health care system. J Manag Care Pharm 2010;16:185–95.

20. Doucette WR, McDonough RP, Klepser D, et al. Comprehensive medication therapy management: identifying and resolving drug-related issues in a community pharmacy. Clin Ther 2005;27:1104–11.

21. Leikola SN, Virolainen J, Tuomainen L, et al. Comprehensive medication reviews for elderly patients: findings and recommendations to physicians. J Am Pharm Assoc 2003;52:630–3.

22. Tse B, Augustine J, Boesen K. Impact of a nationwide medication therapy management program on drug-related problems at the Medication Management Center. 2012. Available at: http://sinfoniarx.com/pdf/Poster.pdf. Accessed May 4, 2016.

23. PhRMA. Improving prescription medicine adherence is key to better health care. 2011. Available at: http://www.phrma.org/sites/default/files/pdf/PhRMA_Improving%20Medication%20Adherence_Issue%20Brief.pdf. Accessed May 4, 2016.

24. Branham A, Moose J, Ferreri S, et al. Retrospective analysis of medication adherence and cost following medication therapy management. Inov Pharm 2010;1(1). Article 12.

25. Cranor CW, Bunting BA, Christensen DB. The Asheville project: long-term outcomes of a community pharmacy diabetes care program. J Am Pharm Assoc 2003;43:183–94.

26. McLean DL, McAlister FA, Johnson JA, et al. A randomized trial of the effect of community pharmacist and nurse care on improving blood pressure management in patients with diabetes mellitus. Arch Intern Med 2008;168:2355–61.

27. Williams AB. Issue brief: medication adherence and health IT. 2014. Available at: http://www.healthit.gov/sites/default/files/medicationadherence_and_hit_issue_brief.pdf. Accessed May 20, 2016.

The Role of Patient Preferences in Deprescribing

Holly M. Holmes, MD, MS[a],*, Adam Todd, PhD, MPharm[b]

KEYWORDS

- Polypharmacy • Inappropriate medication • Deprescribing

KEY POINTS

- With an increasing population with multimorbidity, polypharmacy, and inappropriate medication use, greater focus is being placed on deprescribing as an approach to rationalize medication therapy.
- Deprescribing, generally shown to be feasible and safe, is a process of stopping an inappropriate medication under the supervision of a health care professional.
- Patient preferences should play a central role in deprescribing approaches, particularly in patients for whom deprescribing is a preference-sensitive decision because of uncertainties about the benefits and harms of medications.

INTRODUCTION

The prevalence of polypharmacy continues to increase in the Unites States and elsewhere around the world. With the global aging of the population, clinicians are seeing a shift to a population with comorbidity and subsequent increased medication use. More than half of people more than 65 years of age in the United Stated have 3 or more chronic conditions.[1] In the United States the population greater than 65 years old in 2010 was 13%; by 2030 the older population is projected to reach 20%, whereas, in other developed countries, older people are expected to reach more than 30% of the population by 2030.[2]

Increasing medication use is increasing not only because of higher proportions of older people in the population but also because more and more older people are exposed to polypharmacy. Based on recent US survey data, more than 90% of people 65 years of age and older took at least 1 prescription medication in the prior 30 days, and 39% of older people take 5 or more regular medications on a chronic basis.[3] In the

Disclosure: The authors have nothing to disclose.
[a] Division of Geriatric and Palliative Medicine, UTHealth McGovern Medical School, 6431 Fannin Street, MSB 5.116, Houston, TX 77030, USA; [b] Division of Pharmacy, School of Medicine, Pharmacy and Health, Durham University, C138 Holliday Building, Queen's Campus, Stockton-on-Tees TS176BH, UK
* Corresponding author.
E-mail address: Holly.M.Holmes@uth.tmc.edu

United Kingdom, recent registry data show that 24% of people 80 years of age and older take 10 or more medications regularly.[4]

Although the use of multiple medicines is necessary to treat multiple conditions, taking increasing numbers of medications conveys increasing risks of harm to older patients. Studies of polypharmacy have used different definitions and different methodologies to define the exposure of harmful polypharmacy, and have evaluated different outcomes as measures of harm.[5,6] Despite inconsistencies and heterogeneities in study design, polypharmacy has been shown, primarily in observational studies, to be associated with an increased risk of adverse drug events, hospitalizations, and falls.[7] In addition, the use of multiple medications is associated with an increased likelihood of important therapeutic omissions caused by distraction complexity on the part of clinicians, such as beneficial treatments for heart failure or hypertension.[8] It is unknown whether a reduction in polypharmacy results in improved patient outcomes, but there has been increasing interest in the reduction in medication number as a means to mitigate the harmful effects of polypharmacy.[7]

Given the increasing likelihood that health care providers will be faced with the complexity of care for adults with multimorbidity and the increasing concerns about the harms of polypharmacy, a greater focus has been placed on deprescribing as an approach to rationalizing medication therapy.[9] This article summarizes the definition of deprescribing, reviews the process of deprescribing, discusses the role of patient-centered care in guiding deprescribing interventions, and discusses barriers and possible solutions to deprescribing.

WHAT IS DEPRESCRIBING?

Although many terms have been used to describe the process of stopping medications, including discontinuation, withdrawal, cessation, stopping, and even debridement, the universal use of the term deprescribing has been suggested moving forward to provide consistency.[9,10]

Although there are some variations in the definition of deprescribing, common features include the focus on stopping medications based on lack of benefit or increased risk. Definitions include the cessation of a medication that is no longer necessary,[11] a process of reducing or stopping medications that are harmful or unnecessary,[12] a planned process of stopping medications that are no longer beneficial,[13] and a process of tapering, stopping, discontinuing, or withdrawing drugs.[10] A recent systematic review and network analysis synthesized the various definitions and proposed the following as a definition of deprescribing:

Deprescribing is the process of withdrawal of an inappropriate medication, supervised by a health care professional with the goal of managing polypharmacy and improving outcomes.[10]

The focus of this definition is on deprescribing being a process; as has been previously recommended, the medication use process must integrate prescribing and deprescribing.[14] Medications that are candidates for reduction, by this definition, are inappropriate, which could have different meanings depending on the clinical situation, and are identified based on being high risk, low benefit, or both.

Deprescribing has been shown to be feasible and generally safe, although the possibility of exacerbating the underlying condition being treated should not be discounted, particularly when the condition involves the cardiovascular or central nervous systems.[15,16] A recent systematic review of deprescribing interventions found that it was generally feasible, resulted in reduced medication number, and minimized inappropriate medication use.[17]

THE PROCESS OF DEPRESCRIBING

Basic definitions of deprescribing highlight that simply stopping a medication by not renewing the prescription does not capture the process required to deprescribe. Deprescribing requires a systematic identification of all current medications and prior-itization of medications to be stopped, a determination of the safest means to stop medications, and a monitoring and follow-up plan.[10,18] The 5-step process, proposed by Scott and colleagues,[19] is shown in **Table 1**.

Although the process proposed by Scott and colleagues[21] suggests multiple possible questions to identify drugs that are candidates for deprescribing (step 3 in the process), there are existing tools that could be used in this step. For example, to identify drugs that are contraindicated in certain groups, that have well-known adverse effects, or are either unlikely to cause benefit or the benefit is outweighed by harm, explicit lists such as the Beers criteria or the Screening Tool of Older Persons' Prescrip-tions could be used to determine the drug's eligible for deprescribing.[20,21] Scott and colleagues[19] also propose an algorithm to determine the order and the mode by which medications could be discontinued.

PATIENT PREFERENCES FOR DEPRESCRIBING

The process of deprescribing requires active assessment of patients' attitudes and preferences along the way. For example, patients should be asked whether they think a medication is helpful, whether it is causing side effects or burden and, ultimately, whether they prefer to continue it. Medications that are eligible to be deprescribed and that a patient is willing to stop should be prioritized for deprescribing first, in order to gain patient engagement and trust during the process.[19]

In adults with multimorbidity, in whom benefits and risks of medication therapy are uncertain, and benefits or risks of stopping medications are also uncertain, depres-cribing could be considered a preference-sensitive decision, in which patients' goals and preferences for care should be highly influential in the decision-making process.[1] Identifying medications that are eligible to be deprescribed may be based on an inap-propriate benefit/risk ratio, in addition to the complexity and feasibility of the medica-tion regimen, and the alignment with goals and preferences for care. A proposed framework to identify candidate drugs to stop in such patients is shown in **Fig. 1**.[22]

What do patients think about deprescribing? Few qualitative studies have specif-ically explored patients' attitudes toward deprescribing. A study of the perspectives of long-term care residents and health care professionals suggested that, to be suc-cessful, deprescribing interventions need to take into account the perspectives of mul-tiple stakeholders.[23] For residents in particular, highly ranked concerns included their well-being, continuity of care and communication, the ability to continue medications that contributed to their feeling of wellness, the ability to stop medications they thought to be burdensome, having their voices and rights respected, and respecting the opinions of their physicians.[23] A study of frail long-term care residents and health care professionals in Australia found a significant disconnect between the perceptions of medication benefits on the part of residents and their family members, whereas physicians recognized that, for frail older patients, long-term care was essentially palli-ative.[24] In addition, residents had poor understanding about the indications and possible adverse effects of their medications, low self-efficacy around medication discontinuation, and high trust in their physicians to make medication decisions.[24]

Table 1
The process of deprescribing

Key Step	Detailed Processes
1. Determine all current medications and the indication for each	• Patients should bring all drugs and drug delivery aids to the visit, including over-the-counter drugs and supplements • Ask about adherence in a nonjudgmental way and determine reasons for nonadherence
2. Consider risk of harm in individual patients to determine the intensity of deprescribing	• Determine risk according to drug factors (eg, number of drugs, high-risk drugs) and patient factors (eg, older age, multimorbidity)
3. Assess whether each drug is eligible to be discontinued	• Drugs prescribed for an unconfirmed diagnosis, or drugs not effective for a condition, or drugs that confer no additional benefit after a certain period of use or a certain age • Drugs that are part of a prescribing cascade (prescribed to treat adverse effects of other drugs) • Drugs that are on lists to avoid in older patients • Identify drugs causing well-known adverse effects • Ask patients whether the medicine has made a difference to their symptoms, and whether they would prefer to continue taking it • Ask patients whether a drug is causing any troublesome symptoms • Drugs for self-limiting, mild, or intermittent conditions, or for conditions that respond to nonpharmacologic interventions • Determine the patient's expectations and preferences • Identify drugs unlikely to be of benefit or likely to cause harm in the patient's likely remaining life expectancy • Ask the patient for any other medication-related concerns • Identify burdensome drugs; eg, based on tablet size, cost, monitoring
4. Prioritize drugs for deprescribing	• A possible prioritization for drugs eligible for deprescribing: 1. Drugs that are most harmful and least beneficial 2. Drugs that are easy to stop without likely withdrawal or rebound symptoms 3. Drugs that the patient is most willing to stop
5. Implement and monitor deprescribing regimen	• Discuss plan with patient; reach agreement on the plan • Deprescribe 1 drug at a time • Wean patients off drugs that are likely to cause withdrawal effects • Communicate plan to relevant health care professionals and carers, and/or family involved in patient's care • Fully document the deprescribing plan, including rationale and outcomes

Adapted from Scott IA, Hilmer SN, Reeve E, et al. Reducing inappropriate polypharmacy: the process of deprescribing. JAMA Intern Med 2015;175(5):829.

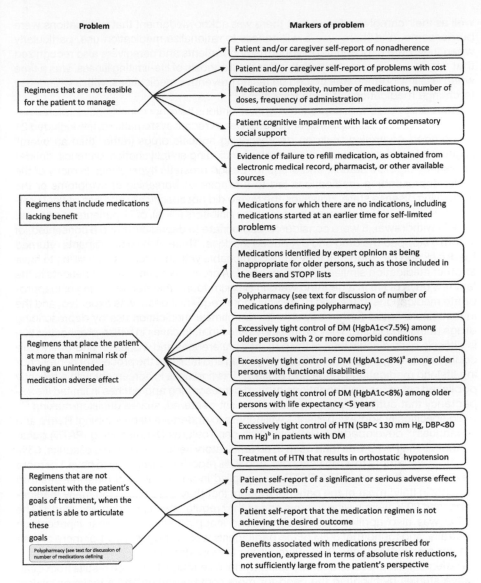

Fig. 1. Strategies for identifying problems with medications: taxonomy of problems with corresponding markers.[a] One panelist provided HgbA1c <7.5%. [b] One panelist provided SBP <140 mm Hg. DBP, diastolic blood pressure; DM, diabetes mellitus; HgbA1c, hemoglobin A1c; HTN, hypertension; SBP, systolic blood pressure. (*From* Fried TR, Niehoff K, Tjia J, et al. A Delphi process to address medication appropriateness for older persons with multiple chronic conditions. BMC Geriatr 2016;16(1):67.)

Similarly, a study of 85 patients with heart failure and 74 prescribing physicians found a disconnect regarding deprescribing; most of the patients were satisfied about the number of medicines they took regularly, and only 41% could identify at least 1 drug they would stop, whereas physicians had a high consensus about drugs that could be stopped when presented with clinical heart failure scenarios.[25] In contrast, a study exploring the medication-related views of patients with life-limiting illness as well as their caregivers found that there was acknowledgment that medications were burdensome, and there was a willingness to rationalize medication use, particularly when they were exposed to polypharmacy.[26] Patients and caregivers also recognized that a transition in care, potentially after the diagnosis of life-limiting illness, was a time when less importance was placed on taking preventive medications, with a willingness to change medications at such transitions.[26]

Trials associated with deprescribing interventions have not consistently explored patient preferences, perceptions, or experiences. A recent systematic review included 21 randomized controlled trials on deprescribing specific drugs (rather than an overall approach to reducing medication number), including antipsychotics, diuretics, antidepressants, digoxin, statins, and drugs for benign prostatic hyperplasia. In many of the trials, deprescribing medications led to a relapse or worsening of symptoms or the underlying disease state. However, the review did not specifically address patient preferences.[16] In a trial of stopping proton pump inhibitors (PPIs), of 72 patients considered for PPI withdrawal, 8 were considered appropriate to deprescribe and 6 consented, of whom 3 stopped the drug and 3 reduced the dose. Three of the 6 participants returned feedback and reported that they were comfortable with the process and willing to have another medication similarly deprescribed.[11] A cross-sectional study of patients in the last few days of life in a geriatric ward in Belgium found that deprescribing of inappropriate medications at the end of life was more frequent if death was expected, and the investigators noted further opportunity to optimize medication use by deprescribing drugs at the end of life. They particularly noted that, in cases in which prognostication is difficult, early discussions of the patient's preferences and wishes for end-of-life care could help to engender trust with the physician and facilitate the process of deprescribing lifelong medications at the end of life.[27] This finding is in agreement with a recently published set of recommendations around deprescribing approaches in limited life expectancy that outline the importance of patient-centered, shared decision-making.[26]

To specifically address patients' willingness to undertake deprescribing, Reeve and colleagues[28] developed the Patients' Attitudes Towards Deprescribing (PATD) questionnaire. The PATD was then used in an ambulatory setting in a sample of adults, 65% of whom were more than 65 years old, and 92% reported willingness to have 1 or more medications stopped.[29] The PATD was applied in a population of older hospitalized patients in Italy; most of the patients thought that they were taking too many medications, and 89% were willing to have one of their regular medicines deprescribed.[30] The PATD was also applied specifically around stopping statins on older inpatients in Australia, and found that 89% of the participants were willing to stop 1 or more of their regular medications, and 95% were willing to stop statins.[31]

Patients' willingness to deprescribe may not be enough. Based on results from qualitative studies highlighting the need for more communication and a focus on patient well-being, and based on quantitative studies showing lower uptake of deprescribing interventions and concerns for relapse of underlying symptoms, a successful deprescribing intervention must seek to fully engage both the patient and, where relevant, the caregiver. The Eliminating Medications Through Patient Ownership of End Results (EMPOWER) trial is an example of such an approach: this intervention was developed to increase patients' knowledge and self-efficacy around stopping benzodiazepines, and was designed to create a cognitive dissonance around the perception that harmful medications were safe.[32] The intervention consisted of a booklet with an assessment about medication risks, education about harms and drug interactions, and a specific stepwise tapering protocol. Overall, 86% completed a 6-month follow-up, at which point 27% of the intervention group had stopped the benzodiazepine, compared with only 5% of the control group (which received general educational materials). This approach has been expanded to other classes of drugs, with publicly available deprescribing algorithms for practitioners to use.[33]

BARRIERS AND PITFALLS TO DEPRESCRIBING

Despite the perceived acceptability of deprescribing and the momentum toward reducing medication use, there are significant barriers to stopping medications. The biggest barrier to deprescribing is an emotional and psychological one: the belief of society and the health care system that every patient-doctor interaction needs to end in the addition of a medication, and that additional medication will either prolong life or promote health.[34] Much has been written about prescribers' discomfort in stopping medications, and emerging discussion of these barriers incorporates a consideration of patient and system barriers to the process.[35] Although there is a disconnect between patients and prescribers regarding the belief about the benefit of medications, the widespread dislike of overmedication is a major enabler of deprescribing as an acceptable intervention.[35] Recent evidence regarding the willingness of patients to stop medications and their reliance on physicians to communicate the need to stop drugs puts the onus back on prescribers to take on responsibility to make deprescribing more commonplace.[18] The barriers to deprescribing are summarized in **Box 1**.

Box 1
Potential barriers to deprescribing

Prescriber

Lack of guidelines, lack of decision support

Lack of time

Fixed beliefs about benefits and harms of medications

Lack of awareness; incomplete medical or medication history

Clinical inertia

Lack of knowledge or skills

Beliefs about external constraints

Need for multiple points of contact/communication to deprescribe

Reluctant to change specialists' medications

Patient

Lack of decision-making capacity

Difficulty in comprehension or communication around deprescribing

Need for caregiver engagement

Misalignment with goals of care

System

Lack of reimbursement

Fragmentation during transitions of care

Lack of facilitators for communication

Absence of integrated electronic medical records system across different sites

Discoordinated care

Data from Refs.[18,23,35–37]

Prescribers' opinions vary widely, particularly about preventive medications, highlighting the need for consensus guidelines around deprescribing.[12] The optimal time at which to deprescribe, the ideal patient situations in which deprescribing should occur, and the ideal settings are unclear and may vary widely based on the individual clinical situation. For example, although transitions of care may represent an ideal time to reconcile and critically rethink all medication therapy, deprescribing in the hospital could be a problem for sustaining change. Deprescribing requires active participation of the patient, including communication and agreement to the change, and acutely ill patients may not be able to participate in deprescribing.[38] Similarly, the ideal patient situations that should prompt deprescribing are uncertain. As an example, patients with dementia may have frequently changing goals of care, making deprescribing necessary as care shifts at the end of life; however, the inability to engage the patient in deprescribing and the need to engage caregivers with frequent communication may present obstacles.[36]

Ultimately, addressing these specific barriers could help to facilitate deprescribing and make stopping medications as facile as prescribing them in the first place. This situation could be accomplished by several changes, which include:

1. Systematically screening patients for their willingness to have medications deprescribed. In much the same way that providers systematically screen for depression or for falls, tools such as the PATD could be used to elicit the patients' attitudes, which could help inform providers about preferences and could facilitate patient-centered decision making about medicines.[28]
2. Providing health information systems that facilitate communication between multiple specialists and with the patient and caregiver, to reduce the concerns about stopping medicines that other prescribers have started.
3. Leveraging data systems to identify medications that are eligible for deprescribing or patients who are ideal candidates for deprescribing interventions.[39] This outcome could be accomplished through the use of existing tools to identify inappropriate medications and tools to identify patients with high-risk conditions.
4. Promoting reimbursement for deprescribing activities by members of a multidisciplinary team, and specifically facilitating the input of pharmacists in making recommendations to deprescribe.
5. Strengthening the evidence based around deprescribing by including patient goal-driven interventions and patient-reported outcomes in deprescribing studies. Future trials of deprescribing should include a qualitative arm if possible, to better understand patients' preferences.

SUMMARY

Deprescribing is more complex than simply stopping medications: it is a multiple-stage process that should be patient centered and a part of the wider remit of shared care decision making.[40] Despite the acknowledgment that patient preferences, alongside those of health care professionals and caregivers, are crucial for any successful deprescribing intervention there is, at present, a dearth of literature in this area. Future studies, particularly randomized controlled trials, should be encouraged to include a qualitative aspect to enable the better understanding of perceptions and experiences for patients who have undergone deprescribing interventions. It will be crucial for future deprescribing interventions to be able to adapt to new evidence as it emerges and still allow for the application of clinical judgment and the consideration of ethical issues.

REFERENCES

1. American Geriatrics Society Expert Panel on the Care of Older Adults with Multi-morbidity. Guiding principles for the care of older adults with multimorbidity: an approach for clinicians. J Am Geriatr Soc 2012;60(10):E1–25.
2. Ortman JM, Velkoff VA, Hogan H. An aging nation: the older population in the United States. US Census Bureau; 2014. p. 25–1140. Available at: https://www.census.gov/prod/2014pubs/p25-1140.pdf. Accessed February 3, 2017.
3. Kantor ED, Rehm CD, Haas JS, et al. Trends in prescription drug use among adults in the United States from 1999-2012. JAMA 2015;314(17):1818–31.
4. Guthrie B, Makubate B, Hernandez-Santiago V, et al. The rising tide of polypharmacy and drug-drug interactions: population database analysis 1995-2010. BMC Med 2015;13:74.
5. Turner JP, Jamsen KM, Shakib S, et al. Polypharmacy cut-points in older people with cancer: how many medications are too many? Support Care Cancer 2016; 24(4):1831–40.
6. Gnjidic D, Hilmer SN, Blyth FM, et al. Polypharmacy cutoff and outcomes: five or more medicines were used to identify community-dwelling older men at risk of different adverse outcomes. J Clin Epidemiol 2012;65(9):989–95.
7. Fried TR, O'Leary J, Towle V, et al. Health outcomes associated with polypharmacy in community-dwelling older adults: a systematic review. J Am Geriatr Soc 2014;62(12):2261–72.
8. Steinman MA, Landefeld CS, Rosenthal GE, et al. Polypharmacy and prescribing quality in older people. J Am Geriatr Soc 2006;54(10):1516–23.
9. Alldred DP. Deprescribing: a brave new word? Int J Pharm Pract 2014;22(1):2–3.
10. Reeve E, Gnjidic D, Long J, et al. A systematic review of the emerging definition of 'deprescribing' with network analysis: implications for future research and clinical practice. Br J Clin Pharmacol 2015;80(6):1254–68.
11. Reeve E, Andrews JM, Wiese MD, et al. Feasibility of a patient-centered deprescribing process to reduce inappropriate use of proton pump inhibitors. Ann Pharmacother 2015;49(1):29–38.
12. Ailabouni NJ, Nishtala PS, Mangin D, et al. General practitioners' insight into deprescribing for the multimorbid older individual: a qualitative study. Int J Clin Pract 2016;70(3):261–76.
13. Potter K, Flicker L, Page A, et al. Deprescribing in frail older people: a randomised controlled trial. PLoS One 2016;11(3):e0149984.
14. Bain KT, Holmes HM, Beers MH, et al. Discontinuing medications: a novel approach for revising the prescribing stage of the medication-use process. J Am Geriatr Soc 2008;56(10):1946–52.
15. Iyer S, Naganathan V, McLachlan AJ, et al. Medication withdrawal trials in people aged 65 years and older: a systematic review. Drugs Aging 2008;25(12): 1021–31.
16. Nguyen T, Gurwitz JH. Deprescribing in older adults: a systematic review. American Geriatrics Society Annual Meeting. Long Beach (CA), May 18–20, 2016.
17. Page AT, Clifford RM, Potter K, et al. The feasibility and the effect of deprescribing in older adults on mortality and health: a systematic review. Br J Clin Pharmacol 2016;82(3):583–623.
18. Scott IA, Le Couteur DG. Physicians need to take the lead in deprescribing. Intern Med J 2015;45(3):352–6.
19. Scott IA, Hilmer SN, Reeve E, et al. Reducing inappropriate polypharmacy: the process of deprescribing. JAMA Intern Med 2015;175(5):827–34.

20. By the American Geriatrics Society Beers Criteria Update Expert Panel. American Geriatrics Society 2015 updated Beers criteria for potentially inappropriate medication use in older adults. J Am Geriatr Soc 2015;63(11):2227–46.

21. O'Mahony D, O'Sullivan D, Byrne S, et al. STOPP/START criteria for potentially inappropriate prescribing in older people: version 2. Age Ageing 2015;44(2): 213–8.

22. Fried TR, Niehoff K, Tjia J, et al. A Delphi process to address medication appropriateness for older persons with multiple chronic conditions. BMC Geriatr 2016; 16(1):67.

23. Turner JP, Edwards S, Stanners M, et al. What factors are important for deprescribing in Australian long-term care facilities? Perspectives of residents and health professionals. BMJ Open 2016;6(3):e009781.

24. Palagyi A, Keay L, Harper J, et al. Barricades and brickwalls–a qualitative study exploring perceptions of medication use and deprescribing in long-term care. BMC Geriatr 2016;16:15.

25. Hopper I, de Silva C, Skiba M, et al. Attitudes of patients and prescribing clinicians to polypharmacy and medication withdrawal in heart failure. J Card Fail 2016;22(9):743–4.

26. Todd A, Holmes H, Pearson S, et al. 'I don't think I'd be frightened if the statins went': a phenomenological qualitative study exploring medicines use in palliative care patients, carers and healthcare professionals. BMC Palliat Care 2016;15:13.

27. Van Den Noortgate NJ, Verhofstede R, Cohen J, et al. Prescription and deprescription of medication during the last 48 hours of life: multicenter study in 23 acute geriatric wards in Flanders, Belgium. J Pain Symptom Manage 2016;51(6): 1020–6.

28. Reeve E, Shakib S, Hendrix I, et al. Development and validation of the patients' attitudes towards deprescribing (PATD) questionnaire. Int J Clin Pharm 2013; 35(1):51–6.

29. Reeve E, Wiese MD, Hendrix I, et al. People's attitudes, beliefs, and experiences regarding polypharmacy and willingness to deprescribe. J Am Geriatr Soc 2013; 61(9):1508–14.

30. Galazzi A, Lusignani M, Chiarelli MT, et al. Attitudes towards polypharmacy and medication withdrawal among older inpatients in Italy. Int J Clin Pharm 2016; 38(2):454–61.

31. Qi K, Reeve E, Hilmer SN, et al. Older peoples' attitudes regarding polypharmacy, statin use and willingness to have statins deprescribed in Australia. Int J Clin Pharm 2015;37(5):949–57.

32. Tannenbaum C, Martin P, Tamblyn R, et al. Reduction of inappropriate benzodiazepine prescriptions among older adults through direct patient education: the EMPOWER cluster randomized trial. JAMA Intern Med 2014;174(6):890–8.

33. Deprescribing algorithms. Available at: deprescribing.org. Accessed May 21, 2016.

34. Garfinkel D, Ilhan B, Bahat G. Routine deprescribing of chronic medications to combat polypharmacy. Ther Adv Drug Saf 2015;6(6):212–33.

35. Reeve E, To J, Hendrix I, et al. Patient barriers to and enablers of deprescribing: a systematic review. Drugs Aging 2013;30(10):793–807.

36. Reeve E, Bell JS, Hilmer SN. Barriers to optimising prescribing and deprescribing in older adults with dementia: a narrative review. Curr Clin Pharmacol 2015;10(3): 168–77.

37. Ailabouni NJ, Nishtala PS, Mangin D, et al. Challenges and enablers of deprescribing: a general practitioner perspective. PLoS One 2016;11(4):e0151066.
38. Ramanathan J. Sustainability of deprescribing post discharge. Intern Med J 2015;45(8):885.
39. Niehoff KM, Rajeevan N, Charpentier PA, et al. Development of the tool to reduce inappropriate medications (TRIM): a clinical decision support system to improve medication prescribing for older adults. Pharmacotherapy 2016;36(6):694–701.
40. Todd A, Holmes HM. Recommendations to support deprescribing medications late in life. Int J Clin Pharm 2015;37(5):678–81.

Polypharmacy Reduction Strategies

Tips on Incorporating American Geriatrics Society Beers and Screening Tool of Older People's Prescriptions Criteria

Hedva Barenholtz Levy, PharmD, BCPS, BCGP

KEYWORDS

- Polypharmacy • Aged/aging • Explicit criteria • Prescribing • Medication use
- Potentially inappropriate medications

KEY POINTS

- Consequences of polypharmacy are numerous and have been associated with negative health outcomes in older adults.
- Several strategies to reduce polypharmacy among older adults have been published that describe various protocols and algorithms.
- The American Geriatrics Society (AGS) Beers Criteria and Screening Tool of Older People's Prescriptions (STOPP) are explicit criteria that address many of the common elements found across these polypharmacy reduction strategies.
- Clinicians can apply components of the AGS Beers and STOPP criteria as a framework for evaluating polypharmacy regimens and reducing polypharmacy.

INTRODUCTION

Aging is associated with increased prevalence of chronic medical conditions and concomitant medication use to manage those conditions. In a recent sampling of community-dwelling older adults in the United States, medication use was associated with both increasing age and number of chronic conditions.[1] More than two-thirds of older adults have at least 2 chronic conditions, and 14% of Medicare beneficiaries manage 6 or more chronic conditions, such as high blood pressure, diabetes, arthritis, or heart failure.[2] In addition, older adults disproportionately consume medications. This age group comprises approximately 13% of the US population, yet accounts

Disclosure: The author received no funding for this article and reports no conflict of interests.
HbL PharmaConsulting, 9648 Olive Boulevard, #309, St Louis, MO 63132, USA
E-mail address: hedva@hblpharm.com

Clin Geriatr Med 33 (2017) 177–187
http://dx.doi.org/10.1016/j.cger.2017.01.007
geriatric.theclinics.com

for 33% of all prescription medication use and 40% of nonprescription medication use.[3]

Increased prevalence of medication use in the US is impressive (**Table 1**).[1,4] Between 1988 and 2010, the median number of prescription medications used by community-dwelling older adults doubled from 2 to 4,[1] with 90% of older adults taking at least 1 prescription medication.[5] These most recent estimates document that 36% to 39% of older adults take 5 or more prescription medications.[1,4] When over-the-counter (OTC) and supplement use is included in medication use estimates, prevalence of older adults taking 5 or more medications increases to 67%.[4] Use of OTC products has declined over time, whereas supplement use has increased, as shown in **Table 1**.[4] Furthermore, older adults frequently combine prescription medications with OTC products and supplements (40% and 66%, respectively), with a concomitant increase in the risk of drug interactions.[4]

As a result of the upward trend in medication use by older adults, clinicians must continue to be increasingly mindful of medication use issues among their older patients. The purpose of this article is to provide an understanding of polypharmacy and its consequences in patient care, review various expert strategies to reduce polypharmacy, and provide suggestions for how to incorporate the 2015 AGS Beers Criteria[6] and STOPP version 2 criteria[7] as part of polypharmacy reduction strategies.

DEFINING POLYPHARMACY

The term, *polypharmacy*, refers to the use of multiple medications and inherently is neutral in meaning. The use of multiple medications, however, typically is associated with clinical and economic consequences (summarized later). As a result, the term polypharmacy has come to be associated with a negative connotation by most clinicians.

There is no single accepted definition of polypharmacy. It can be defined either numerically or in a qualitative manner. The numeric definition can vary by practice setting or research protocol. Commonly, polypharmacy is defined in the literature as the use of 5 or more medications. Often, a numeric-based definition is considered too simplistic, because the number of medications alone is not always problematic.[8] Drug therapy that has been optimized for a particular patient, is evidence-based, has appropriate indications for use, and is carefully monitored with achievement of desired health outcomes could be considered appropriate polypharmacy.

Table 1 Trends in medication use among older adults		
	1988	2010
Use of ≥5 prescription medications, persons age 65 and older (Charlesworth et al,[1] 2015)	13%	39%
	2005	2011
Use of ≥5 prescription medications, persons 62–85 y (Qato et al,[4] 2016)	31%	36%
Use of ≥1 OTC medications, persons 62–85 y (Qato et al,[4] 2016)	44%	38%
Use of ≥1 supplements, persons 62–85 y (Qato et al,[4] 2016)	52%	64%

Data from Charlesworth CJ, Smit E, Lee DSH, et al. Polypharmacy among adults aged 65 years and older in the United States: 1988–2010. J Gerontol A Biol Sci Med Sci 2015;70:989–95; and Qato DM, Wilder J, Schumm P, et al. Changes in prescription and over-the-counter medication and dietary supplement use among older adults in the United States, 2005 vs. 2011. JAMA Intern Med 2016;176:475–82.

Therefore, qualitative definitions of polypharmacy are helpful. To this end, polypharmacy has been defined as the use of multiple unnecessary medications, the use of more medications than are clinically warranted or indicated, or the use of unnecessary, ineffective, or harmful prescribing.[8–10] This qualitative approach frames polypharmacy in a negative manner that alludes to the adverse outcomes associated with medication use. To help clinicians identify patients at higher risk of medication-related problems, it has been suggested that problematic polypharmacy should be differentiated from appropriate polypharmacy and that consideration of overall appropriateness of therapy is more valuable than simply considering the number of medications an older person is prescribed.[11]

In this article, polypharmacy refers to problematic or inappropriate polypharmacy. When defined in this manner, polypharmacy reduction strategies encompass both reducing the number of medications prescribed (eg, discontinuing medications that are without an indication or are harmful) and addressing unnecessary and ineffective prescribing. Thus, understanding polypharmacy in both a quantitative and qualitative manner allows clinicians to consider a more comprehensive approach to addressing problems related to polypharmacy.

CONSEQUENCES OF POLYPHARMACY

Polypharmacy can have myriad negative effects on quality of patient care and health outcomes. Several articles have reviewed the evidence supporting consequences of polypharmacy. The most commonly cited consequences are listed in **Box 1**.[3,12–15] The risk of adverse drug reactions due to polypharmacy is interrelated with increased prescribing of potentially inappropriate medications (PIMs).[15,16] PIMs are widely associated with negative health outcomes.[17] It is not surprising, therefore, that polypharmacy reduction strategies almost universally include a component to address the presence of high-risk or harmful prescribing in polypharmacy regimens.

POLYPHARMACY REDUCTION STRATEGIES

Several tools have been described for use in the elderly population that are designed to educate and guide clinicians in efforts to reduce polypharmacy.[18,19] These various tools can be categorized as implicit-based and explicit-based approaches. The implicit-based approaches by definition are judgment based and rely on clinical

---

Box 1
Consequences of polypharmacy

- Increased risk of adverse drug reactions
- Reduced medication adherence
- Increased risk of serious drug-drug interactions
- Increased health care costs
- Reduced functional ability and ability to perform independent activities of daily living
- Increased risk of geriatric syndromes, such as
  - Cognitive impairment
  - Falls
  - Malnutrition
  - Urinary incontinence

Data from Refs.[3,12–15]

information for interpretation and assessment. In contrast, explicit-based approaches, such as AGS Beers[6] and STOPP/Screening Tool to Alert to Right Treatment (START),[7] require no or minimal clinical judgment to interpret.

Many of the implicit-based approaches are protocols or algorithms designed to streamline the medication review process. Some of these approaches focus specifically on deprescribing or reducing the number of prescribed drugs.[20–23] Others present conceptual or philosophic guidelines to promote a more judicious approach to prescribing in this age group.[3,24–26] By nature, these approaches are highly individualized and rely on the clinician's experience and assessment. They are thus more challenging to apply in a consistent manner across patient populations.

Two examples of systematic approaches to optimize polypharmacy are summarized in **Table 2**.[10,12] Both protocols are designed for use in older adults. The Assess, Review, Minimize, Optimize, Reassess (ARMOR) protocol was developed for the long-term care setting, but the investigators encourage its use in the outpatient setting as well. Application of the tool has not been rigorously studied, but it was associated with reduced number of medications prescribed, falls, and hospitalization in their study population.[10] The Prescribing Optimization Method (POM) was developed to provide general practitioners with a rapid and easy tool to optimize prescribing in older adults in the community.[12] Application of the POM significantly increased the frequency of appropriate drug therapy decisions made by general practitioners and improved underuse of medications. General practitioners who used the POM had greater concordance of prescribing decisions compared with geriatric experts.

Common core elements are shared by the several implicit-based tools to optimize polypharmacy:

- Define or confirm clinical indications for all medications a patient takes.
- Adjust dosages for renal function.
- Assess relative risks and benefits of each medication; identify adverse drug events.
- Evaluate drug interactions, including both drug-drug and drug-condition interactions.

Assessment of the relative risks and benefits of medications and adverse drug events is an element that appears almost uniformly across the implicit-based protocols and algorithms. The core elements, identified previously, are directly related to the explicit criteria. Thus, a discussion of ways to incorporate the AGS Beers and STOPP into polypharmacy reduction strategies is warranted.

INCORPORATING EXPLICIT CRITERIA INTO POLYPHARMACY REDUCTION STRATEGIES
American Geriatrics Society Beers and Screening Tool of Older People's Prescriptions

Two of the most widely accepted explicit criteria are the AGS Beers[6] and STOPP/START.[7] Although they share some common content, they each have unique characteristics that are important for clinicians to appreciate.[17] By definition, explicit criteria are more objective than implicit criteria and easier to apply in a consistent manner to the medication review process.[27] AGS Beers and STOPP are tools that can be applied in different ways to improve polypharmacy. They can serve as research tools to measure prevalence of or changes in appropriateness of therapy.[11] They also can be applied as clinical tools to improve the quality of prescribing and ideally clinical outcomes for older adults. The START criteria address omissions of therapy, which are an important factor in problematic polypharmacy.[16] Addressing drug therapy omissions is an integral component of optimizing polypharmacy in older adults and should

Table 2 Systematic approaches to address polypharmacy		
Polypharmacy Strategy	**Overview**	**Description**
ARMOR[10]	Acronym stands for Assess, Review, Minimize, Optimize, Reassess	Assess all medications, including β_1-blockers, pain medications, psychotropics, other medications on the Beers criteria, and vitamins and supplements. Review for drug-drug and drug-disease interactions and adverse drug reactions. Minimize the number of medications according to functional status rather than evidence-based medicine; minimize nonessential medications. Optimize drug therapy for renal or hepatic clearance and targeted biologic or pharmacodynamic response markers (heart rate, serum drug levels, etc.); consider gradual dose reduction for antidepressants; avoid therapy duplications. Reassess patient for functional and cognitive status, clinical status, and medication adherence.
Prescribing Optimization Method[12]	Consists of 6 questions that could be asked by general practitioners or members of a multidisciplinary team	1. Is patient undertreated and is additional medication indicated? 2. Does patient adhere to medication schedule? 3. Which drugs can be withdrawn and which are inappropriate for patient? 4. Which adverse effects are present? 5. What clinically relevant interactions are to be expected? 6. Should dose frequency or form of the drug be adjusted?

Data from Haque R. ARMOR: a tool to evaluate polypharmacy in elderly persons. Ann Long-Term Care 2009;17(6):26–30; and Drenth-van Maanen AC, van Marum RJ, Knol W, et al. Prescribing optimization method for improving prescribing in elderly patients receiving polypharmacy. Drugs Aging 2009;26(8):687–701.

be included in any such endeavors. This article focuses, however, on PIM use and application of AGS Beers and STOPP.

Tips for Incorporating the Explicit Criteria

Key principles for how to use the AGS Beers have been delineated.[28] First and foremost, the drugs and drug classes on the list are potentially inappropriate, not definitely inappropriate. The medications on these lists may be an appropriate choice for certain patients in certain situations. Subsequently, clinicians need to understand both the rationale and recommendations that accompany each of the AGS Beers criteria and think through why the drug or drug class is included. For STOPP, indicators contain an explanation and references with which clinicians should be familiar. Importantly, AGS Beers and STOPP are educational tools designed to encourage clinicians to pause and reflect on risks and benefits of certain medications before prescribing them or to be more vigilant to possible adverse drug reactions. The criteria are not all encompassing of medication-related problems in older adults; for example, they do not address many implicit considerations like drug effectiveness, adverse effects, or adherence. As such, they should be viewed as an entry point to more comprehensive medication reviews.

Ideally, clinicians would conduct a medication review by screening all the explicit criteria against a patient's polypharmacy regimen. The 2 sets of criteria, however, are lengthy and with many nuances. Thus, a more focused approach to using the explicit criteria might be more practical, for example, based on key concepts that are common to both sets of explicit criteria. A framework for how the AGS Beers and STOPP can be incorporated into a polypharmacy reduction strategy is described (see also **Table 3**).[6,7,29]

1. Define or confirm clinical indications for all medications a patient takes. STOPP includes an indicator that specifies "Any drug prescribed without an evidence-based clinical indication" as a potentially inappropriate prescribing situation in older adults.[7] This is 1 of 3 implicit criteria that are included among the 81 total indicators in STOPP. AGS Beers does not contain a similar criterion. This most fundamental aspect of addressing polypharmacy warrants its inclusion as an aspect of the explicit criteria, even though it appears only in STOPP.

2. Adjust dosages for renal function. In their most recent updates, both AGS Beers and STOPP added specific sections dedicated to high-risk medications that need to be dose adjusted or avoided based on renal function. AGS Beers added a new table; STOPP added a separate category. Both lists exclude mention of anti-infective agents, with the exception of nitrofurantoin, which is mentioned in AGS Beers.[6] These lists are not all inclusive but specify the most important drugs for which dosage adjustment or avoidance is deemed critical to their safe prescribing. There is limited overlap between the drugs identified by AGS Beers and STOPP, with only the direct-acting oral anticoagulants and colchicine appearing in both sets of criteria in the dedicated renal function–focused portions of the criteria. **Table 3** compares other medications found in either of the criteria.

3. Evaluate drug-drug interactions. Non–anti-infective drug-drug interactions are included in both criteria. The 2015 AGS Beers contains a new table dedicated to serious drug-drug interactions. In contrast, clinically pertinent drug-drug interactions are interspersed throughout the STOPP indicators. The drug-drug interactions included in the criteria are not comprehensive but are selectively identified due to high risk of harms in older adults. To fully evaluate drug interactions, clinicians must refer to more complete references and databases. Drug-drug interactions that are found in both AGS Beers and STOPP include:

   ○ Combinations of drugs that increase the risk of bleeding or gastrointestinal ulcers (eg, warfarin, direct-acting oral anticoagulants, antiplatelet agents, aspirin, and corticosteroids)
   ○ Drugs that interact with angiotensin-converting enzyme inhibitors and/or otherwise increase serum potassium levels

4. Evaluate drug-disease or syndrome interactions. AGS Beers contains a table of 12 different conditions with recommendations regarding PIMs for each situation.[6]

Table 3
Tips for incorporating the American Geriatrics Society Beers and Screening Tool of Older People's Prescriptions criteria to reduce polypharmacy

Drug Therapy Issue	Comments
Check for clinical indication for all medications.	This implicit indicator is found only in STOPP.
Check for medications that require dose adjustment because of renal elimination.	Digoxin, NSAIDs, direct-acting oral anticoagulants, and colchicine are common to both sets of criteria. Examples of additional agents found in AGS Beers are histamine$_2$-receptor antagonists, duloxetine, gabapentin, and spironolactone. Metformin appears only in STOPP. The criteria differ in their creatinine clearance thresholds for specific medications, so regionally accepted dosing guidelines should be considered.
Check for drug-drug interactions.	AGS Beers drug interaction table contains interactions with warfarin and lithium, along with several other pharmacokinetic and pharmacodynamics drug interactions. Fewer drug-drug interactions are found in STOPP; they are interspersed throughout the indicators.
Check for drug-disease or syndrome interactions.	Drug-disease interactions mentioned in both sets of criteria are numerous. AGS Beers and STOPP share some overlap, with many other drug-disease interactions found only in 1 set of criteria or the other.
Evaluate potentially inappropriate medications based on risk:benefit assessment.	Medications included in AGS Beers and STOPP are PIMs and thus have high risk:benefit ratio. Clinicians need to carefully read the rationale and recommendations provided in AGS Beers and the complete explanation of each indicator as written in STOPP to understand the reason for including various PIMs. Exceptions to the criteria are provided for many of the PIMs on these lists.
Consider duration of use.	Common to both lists are PPIs and NSAIDs. STOPP also mentions corticosteroids, BZDs (note that AGS Beers does not recommend BZDs for any duration of use) and anticoagulants for treatment of DVT and PE.
Check for duplication of medications.	Consider anticholinergic agents and central nervous system-active agents as well as duplicate drugs from the same drug class, for example, NSAIDs, SSRIs, etc.
Identify opportunities to promote nonpharmacologic treatments.	Conditions for which there are evidence-based nonpharmacologic approaches[29]: Appetite Delirium and behavioral and psychological symptoms of dementia Pain Sleep Urinary incontinence

Abbreviations: DVT, deep vein thrombosis; PE, pulmonary embolism; PPIs, proton pump inhibitors; SSRIs, selective serotonin reuptake inhibitors.
   Data from Refs.[6,7,29]

STOPP indicators frequently are based on drug use related to a medical condition, and thus drug-disease interaction indicators are interspersed throughout the indicator list. Consequently, clinicians need to peruse all of the STOPP criteria to glean the various drug-disease interactions identified. Diseases or syndromes that appear in both sets of criteria are summarized, along with interacting drugs or characteristics that are recommended to be avoided or require greater scrutiny. The published criteria contain more specific drug information.

- Heart failure – drugs that increase fluid retention or exacerbate heart failure (eg, verapamil, diltiazem, nonsteroidal anti-inflammatory drugs [NSAIDs], thiazolidinediones)
- Syncope or bradycardia – drugs that increase orthostatic hypotension or bradycardia (eg, acetylcholinesterase inhibitors and α_1-blockers)
- Delirium and dementia or cognitive impairment – antipsychotics and drugs with anticholinergic properties
- History of falls or high risk for falls – drugs that affect gait, balance, orthostatic hypotension (eg, benzodiazepines [BZDs], non-BZDs, and antipsychotics are mentioned in both criteria)
- Parkinson disease – drugs that are dopamine receptor antagonists
- Peptic ulcer disease or history of gastrointestinal bleeding – drugs that are gastric irritants (ie, aspirin and NSAIDs)
- Urinary incontinence – drugs that aggravate or exacerbate urinary incontinence (eg, estrogen, α_1-blockers,[6] and furosemide to treat hypertension[7])
- Lower urinary tract symptoms/benign prostatic hyperplasia – drugs that increase urinary retention (eg, strongly anticholinergic drugs)

Many additional drug-disease interactions are found exclusively in either AGS Beers or STOPP; thus readers are referred directly to each of the published criteria.[6,7]

5. Evaluate relative risks and benefits of each medication; identify medications for which risks exceed clinical benefit. This component by definition essentially encompasses all of the AGS Beers and STOPP criteria, because PIMs are defined as medications for which the risks generally outweigh benefits. Examples of drugs or drug classes that are considered PIMs by both sets of criteria are listed and represent medications that deserve careful scrutiny when prescribed for older adults. Readers are referred to the complete updated published criteria for a comprehensive view of PIMs and associated explanations.[6,7]

- Anticholinergic drugs
- Antipsychotic drugs
- BZDs and non-BZDs
- Methyltestosterone and testosterone
- Estrogen
- Long-acting sulfonylureas
- NSAIDs, both selective and nonselective

Additional drugs or drug classes are included in the criteria because of questionable effectiveness in addition to risk of adverse drug events (eg, antispasmodics and skeletal muscle relaxants).[6] Other medications are identified as PIMs only in certain situations. Thus, careful perusal of the rationale and recommendations in AGS Beers and the complete indicators in STOPP is warranted. Some medications, for example, are recommended to be avoided as first-line choices but could be appropriate if other options fail, such as with amiodarone for atrial fibrillation or centrally acting antihypertensive agents for hypertension.[6,7]

6. Evaluate appropriate duration of use for medicines with evidence-based defined parameters. In addition to the medications specifically mentioned in the criteria (see **Table 3**), "Any drug prescribed beyond the recommended duration, where treatment duration is well defined" is an implicit criterion in STOPP.[7]
7. Check for drug duplication. This is another of the 3 implicit criteria found in STOPP: "Any duplicate drug class prescription."[7] In addition, both sets of criteria specifically mention avoiding combination of 2 or more anticholinergic drugs. AGS Beers mentions avoiding the use of 3 or more central nervous system–active drugs.[6]
8. Promote nonpharmacologic therapies when appropriate. Interest in identifying evidence-based support for nonpharmacologic treatments is growing.[29,30] Both sets of criteria state that nonpharmacologic treatment of behavioral symptoms of dementia or delirium is preferred over antipsychotic agents due to stroke and mortality risk. A companion article to the AGS Beers references evidence-based nonpharmacologic approaches that are alternatives to medications in the AGS Beers list.[29]

LIMITATIONS TO USING THE EXPLICIT CRITERIA

Limitations of using the explicit criteria to review for polypharmacy issues must be emphasized. AGS Beers and STOPP cannot evaluate adherence, drug therapy omission, patient preferences, and issues related to comorbidities, for example. Thus the explicit criteria should not be applied in isolation of a more comprehensive approach that addresses these and other components of optimal medication use. Furthermore, the drugs and drug classes included in the criteria are considered potentially inappropriate; certain PIMs could be appropriate depending on an individual patient's situation.

In addition, many of the polypharmacy optimization strategies laid out by various experts include components that cannot be addressed by the explicit criteria; for example, dose reduction is commonly included in these strategies. Dose adjusting for renal function is addressed by the explicit criteria, as described previously. However, another opportunity to reduce dosages is in patients for whom less stringent treatment targets are appropriate, such as diabetes or blood pressure targets in patients with comorbidities or limited longevity.[31–34]

Finally, the criteria are increasingly complex and require some level of clinical data for assessment. The 2015 AGS Beers added 2 major tables to its criteria: drug-drug interactions and kidney function considerations.[6] The newest version also includes more exceptions to certain criteria. STOPP version 2 is expanded by 31% over the original version.[7] Its indicators typically include clinical scenarios that delineate specific conditions in which a medication is considered inappropriate. Consequently, additional clinical information is needed to fully assess many of these indicators. Thus a simple checklist is challenging to create. Computerized support programs that adapt these or other approaches are being explored to improve quality of prescribing in older adults.[35,36]

SUMMARY

Polypharmacy and its attendant consequences have far-reaching implications in health care for the older adult population. Several protocols and algorithms to optimize polypharmacy have been developed that share common core elements. Implicit or judgment-based approaches can be difficult to apply with consistency, because they inherently require clinical interpretation. The AGS Beers and STOPP criteria are tools that also can be used to improve polypharmacy, either as part of these approaches or independently. Unifying concepts found in both AGS Beers and STOPP can serve as a framework for clinicians to incorporate the explicit criteria into polypharmacy reduction strategies.

REFERENCES

1. Charlesworth CJ, Smit E, Lee DSH, et al. Polypharmacy among adults aged 65 years and older in the United States: 1988-2010. J Gerontol A Biol Sci Med Sci 2015;70:989–95.
2. Centers for Medicare and Medicaid Services (CMS). Chronic conditions among Medicare beneficiaries, Chartbook, 2012 edition. Baltimore (MD): CMS; 2012.
3. Shah BM, Hajjar ER. Polypharmacy, adverse drug reactions, and geriatric syndromes. Clin Geriatr Med 2012;28:173–86.
4. Qato DM, Wilder J, Schumm P, et al. Changes in prescription and over-the-counter medication and dietary supplement use among older adults in the United States, 2005 vs. 2011. JAMA Intern Med 2016;176:475–82.
5. Kantor ED, Rehm CD, Haas JS, et al. Trends in prescription drug use among adults in the United States from 1999-2012. J Am Med Assoc 2015;314:1818–31.
6. American Geriatrics Society 2015 Beers Criteria Update Expert Panel. American Geriatrics Society 2015 updated Beers Criteria for potentially inappropriate medication use in older adults. J Am Geriatr Soc 2015;63:2227–46.
7. O'Mahony D, O'Sullivan D, Byrne S, et al. STOPP/START criteria for potentially inappropriate prescribing in older people: version 2. Age Ageing 2015;44:213–8.
8. Steinman MA. Polypharmacy—time to get beyond numbers. JAMA Intern Med 2016;176:482–3.
9. Rollason V, Vogt N. Reduction of polypharmacy in the elderly, a systematic review of the role of the pharmacist. Drugs Aging 2003;20:817–32.
10. Haque R. ARMOR: a tool to evaluate polypharmacy in elderly persons. Ann Long-Term Care 2009;17(6):26–30.
11. Patterson SM, Cadogan CA, Kerse N, et al. Interventions to improve the appropriate use of polypharmacy for older people (review). Cochrane Database Syst Rev 2014;(10):CD008165.
12. Drenth-van Maanen AC, van Marum RJ, Knol W, et al. Prescribing optimization method for improving prescribing in elderly patients receiving polypharmacy. Drugs Aging 2009;26(8):687–701.
13. Maher RL, Hanlon JT, Hajjar ER. Clinical consequences of polypharmacy in elderly. Expert Opin Drug Saf 2014;13(1):57–65.
14. Doan J, Zakrewski-Jakubiak H, Roy J, et al. Prevalence and risk of potential cytrochrome P450-mediated drug-drug interactions in older hospitalized patients with polypharmacy. Ann Pharmacother 2013;47(3):324–32.
15. Hajjar ER, Cafiero AC, Hanlon JT. Polypharmacy in elderly patients. Am J Geriatr Pharmacother 2007;5:345–51.
16. Steinman MA, Landefeld CS, Rosenthal GE, et al. Polypharmacy and prescribing quality in older people. J Am Geriatr Soc 2006;54:1516–23.
17. Levy HB, Marcus EL. Potentially inappropriatekk medications in older adults: why the revised criteria matter. Ann Pharmacother 2016;50(7):599–603.
18. Frank C, Weir E. Deprescribing for older patients. CMAJ 2014;186(18):1369–76.
19. Gokula M, Holmes HM. Tools to reduce polypharmacy. Clin Geriatr Med 2012;28:323–41.
20. Courtney DL. Medication reduction strategies. Compr Ther 1996;22:318–23.

21. Garfinkel D, Zur-Gil S, Ben-Israel J. The war against polypharmacy: a new cost-effective geriatric-palliative approach for improving drug therapy in disabled elderly people. Isr Med Assoc J 2007;9:430–4.
22. Garfinkel D, Mangin D. Feasibility study of a systematic approach for discontinuation of multiple medications in older adults. Arch Intern Med 2010;170: 1648–54.
23. Scott IA, Hilmer SN, Reeve E. Reducing inappropriate polypharmacy, the process of deprescribing. JAMA Intern Med 2015;175:827–34.
24. Schiff GD, Galanter WL, Duhig J, et al. Principles of conservative prescribing. Arch Intern Med 2011;171:1433–40.
25. Scott IA, Gray LC, Martin JH, et al. Minimizing inappropriate medications in older populations: a 10-step conceptual framework. Am J Med 2012;125:529–37.
26. Sönnichsen A, Trampisch US, Rieckert A, et al. Polypharmacy in chronic diseases—reduction of inappropriate medication and adverse drug events in older populations by electronic decision support (PRIMA-eDS): study protocol for a randomized controlled trial. Trials 2016;17:57.
27. Spinewine A, Schmader KE, Barber N, et al. Appropriate prescribing in elderly people: how well can it be measured and optimised? Lancet 2007;370(9582): 173–84.
28. Steinman MA, Beizer JL, DuBeau CE, et al. How to use the American Geriatrics Society 2015 Beers Criteria—a guide for patients, clinicians, health systems, and payors. J Am Geriatr Soc 2015;63(2):e1–8.
29. Hanlon JT, Semla TP, Schmader KE. Alternative medications for medications in the use of high-risk medications in the elderly and potentially harmful drug-disease interactions in the elderly quality measures. J Am Geriatr Soc 2015; 63(2):e8–18.
30. Abraha I, Cruz-Jentoft A, Soiza RL, et al. Evidence of and recommendations for non-pharmacological interventions for common geriatric conditions: the SENATOR-ONTOP systematic review protocol. BMJ Open 2015;5:e007488.
31. Tseng CL, Soroka O, Maney M, et al. Assessing potential glycemic overtreatment in persons at hypoglycemic risk. JAMA Intern Med 2014;174(2):259–68.
32. Byatt K. Overenthusiastic stroke risk factor modification in the over-80s: are we being disingenuous to ourselves, and to our oldest patients? Evid Based Med 2014;19(4):121–2.
33. Sussman JB, Kerr EA, Saini SD, et al. Rates of deintensification of blood pressure and glycemic medication treatment based on levels of control and life expectancy in older patients with diabetes mellitus. JAMA Intern Med 2015;175(12): 1942–9.
34. Lipska KJ, Ross JS, Miao Y, et al. Potential overtreatment of diabetes mellitus in older adults with tight glycemic control. JAMA Intern Med 2015;175(3):356–62.
35. Meulendijk MC, Spruit MR, Drenth-van Maanen AC, et al. Computerized decision support improves medication review effectiveness: an experiment evaluating the STRIP assistant's usability. Drugs Aging 2015;32:495–503.
36. Bjerre LM, Halil R, Catley C, et al. Potentially inappropriate prescribing (PIP) in long-term care (LTC) patients: validation of the 2014 STOPP-START and 2012 Beers criteria in a LTC population-a protocol for cross-sectional comparison of clinical and health administrative data. BMJ Open 2015;5(10):e009715.

Polypharmacy and Delirium in Critically Ill Older Adults
Recognition and Prevention

Erik Garpestad, MD[a], John W. Devlin, PharmD[a,b],*

KEYWORDS

- Polypharmacy • Delirium • Medications • Older adults • Intensive care
- Antipsychotic agents • Benzodiazepine • Prevention

KEY POINTS

- Polypharmacy is a common sequelae of ICU admissions and is associated with increased medication-associated adverse events, drug interactions, and health care costs.
- Delirium is prevalent in critically ill older adults and medications, many of which are commonly administered in the ICU, remain important modifiable risk factors for delirium in this setting.
- The medication list for a patient with delirium should be carefully reviewed and drugs known to potentiate delirium should be stopped or replaced with a medication not known to induce delirium.
- In patients with delirium, nonpharmacologic interventions, such as early mobilization, should be tried before medications such as antipsychotics given the much stronger evidence supporting their use.
- The incorporation of critical care pharmacists on ICU rounds and implementation of formal medication reconciliation efforts are important strategies to reduce polypharmacy in older adults who develop delirium while admitted to the ICU.

INTRODUCTION

Polypharmacy is common among critically ill older adults and is associated with increased adverse events, greater drug interactions, and increased costs. Delirium occurs in more than half of older adults admitted to the intensive care unit (ICU) and is associated with well-recognized short- and long-term adverse outcomes. Several medications, many of which are routinely used in the critically ill, are specific

Conflict of Interest: None of the authors declare conflicts of interest surrounding this article.
[a] Division of Pulmonary, Critical Care, and Sleep Medicine, Tufts Medical Center, 200 Washington Street, Boston, MA 02111, USA; [b] School of Pharmacy, Northeastern University, 360 Huntington Avenue 140TF RD218F, Boston, MA 02115, USA
* Corresponding author. School of Pharmacy, Northeastern University, 360 Huntington Avenue 140TF RD218F, Boston, MA 02115.
E-mail address: j.devlin@neu.edu

Clin Geriatr Med 33 (2017) 189–203
http://dx.doi.org/10.1016/j.cger.2017.01.002
0749-0690/17/© 2017 Elsevier Inc. All rights reserved.

geriatric.theclinics.com

modifiable risk factors for delirium in this population. Pharmacologic ICU delirium treatment interventions, particularly antipsychotics, may contribute to polypharmacy during and after the ICU stay. This article reviews the literature on polypharmacy and delirium, with a particular focus on the causal relationship between polypharmacy and delirium in critically ill, older adults. Offered are clinician strategies on how to recognize and reduce medication-associated delirium and recommendations on how to reduce or prevent polypharmacy in a patient who develops delirium.

POLYPHARMACY IN CRITICALLY ILL OLDER ADULTS

Older adults (≥65 years) compromise an ever-increasing proportion of patients admitted to the ICU.[1] Very old adults (≥80 years) make up more than 25% of the patients admitted to the ICU; the rate of admission of this population is expected to increase by 6% per year during the next decade. Advanced age is associated with increased ICU mortality and greater post-ICU morbidity.[2] The number of chronically critically ill older adults who are cared for in long-term acute care hospitals, and frequently transition between the long-term acute care hospitals and ICU setting, also continues to increase.[3]

Older adults who are admitted to the ICU take an average of 12 different prescription medications at the time of admission.[4] Among older adults, adverse drug events account for more than 30% of all hospital admissions and specific drug-related causes are a common reason for entry to the ICU.[5,6] Over the past decade, older adults have doubled their use of herbal and over-the-counter medications; 15% experience a major herbal/over-the-counter prescription drug interaction each year.[7] Prescribing cascades (ie, where a new medication is initiated to treat the side effect of another) remains an additional driver of polypharmacy in the critical care setting.

Safe and effective medication use is crucial to ensure optimal patient care and ICU outcome. Furthermore, the acute organ dysfunction prevalent during critical illness may affect drug absorption, clearance, and response, and therefore increase adverse events.[8] However, the complexity and severity that characterizes critical illness, coupled with evidence gaps and features unique to the ICU setting, makes the judicious use of medication in this setting often challenging. Moreover, data generated in non-ICU settings may not transpose to the ICU where patient acuity is higher, goals of therapy are different (and frequently change), duration of medication use is usually short, and monitoring practices are more rigorous.[9] The dearth of rigorous data to guide prescribing decisions for the critically ill results in "off-label" use for nearly half the medications ultimately prescribed in the ICU.[10]

Several drugs often used to treat critical illness are listed in the Beers inventory of low benefit and/or high-risk medications, a medication list deemed by geriatricians as preferably avoided in older adults in chronic health care settings.[11] Potentially inappropriate medications are frequently prescribed in the ICU setting[12]; the number of potentially inappropriate medications prescribed directly correlates with the duration of the ICU stay.[13] Factors associated with an increased risk for a potentially inappropriate medication being continued at ICU discharge include the number of potentially inappropriate medications prescribed at ICU admission, an admission to a surgical (vs medical) service, and discharge to another facility (vs home).[14]

Transitions of care (ie, when a patient moves across different care sites in the health system) are frequent among older adults. This population often resides in long-term care and during periods of decompensation or a new acute illness requires management in an acute care setting that may include an ICU. During these transitions, patients are vulnerable and medication errors, either through drug additions or omissions, may lead to adverse events. Strategies that improve continuity of care, minimize care gaps and foster better communication between clinicians will reduce medication error and improve outcome.[15] Complex hospitalized patients, many of which spend some part of their stay in an ICU, are at a particularly high risk for errors during each care transition and experiencing adverse drug events related to polypharmacy-associated drug–drug interactions.[16]

DELIRIUM IN CRITICALLY ILL OLDER ADULTS

Delirium is a syndrome characterized by the acute onset of cerebral dysfunction with a change or fluctuation in baseline mental status, inattention, and either disorganized thinking or an altered level of consciousness.[17] Other symptoms commonly associated with delirium include sleep disturbances, abnormal psychomotor activity, hallucinations, delusions, and emotional disturbance (eg, fear, anxiety, anger, depression, apathy, and euphoria).[18] These latter sequelae are often the symptoms that are most concerning to patients, family members, and caregivers.

Age is one of the most important underlying risk factors for delirium. More than a third of older adults have delirium at the time of ICU admission.[19] Although studies from 15 years ago report a delirium prevalence of 80% in older adults who require mechanical ventilator support, the current rate of delirium in this population is closer to 50% given the far greater number of patients who are now managed at a light level of sedation and mobilized early.[19,20] The prevalence of delirium remains high; a greater focus on the importance of polypharmacy as a cause for delirium may help reduce it.

Delirium as a manifestation of acute brain dysfunction is associated with several undesirable ICU outcomes including self-extubation, a longer duration of mechanical ventilation, and greater long-term mortality.[20] Older adults who develop delirium in the ICU are more likely to transition to a skilled nursing facility (eg, nursing home) than a rehabilitation facility or home.[20] Delirium may lead to cognitive impairment 6 months after ICU discharge similar in severity to that observed with moderate dementia or after traumatic brain injury.[21] These cognitive deficits often persist for weeks or months (or never resolve at all) and often prevent the ability of patients to resume precritical illness activities and function. The burden of delirium can have profound effects on spouses and family members, particularly if they are required to assume a caregiver role on a persistent basis.[20] With the effects of delirium often persisting long after the ICU discharge, it is now recognized to be a major public health problem in the United States that costs more than $15 billion each year.[22]

Delirium is challenging to recognize in the ICU setting because most patients are intubated and cannot verbally communicate, medications that reduce the level of consciousness are used prevalently, hypoactive delirium is common, and patients may be too unstable to participate in lengthy assessments.[23] The ability to recognize delirium accurately is a key component when developing interprofessional strategies focused on reducing reversible causes and initiating appropriate treatment strategies.[22] Among the ICU delirium screening tools developed, the Confusion Assessment Method for the ICU and the Intensive Care Delirium Screening Checklist are the two instruments that have the greatest psychometric strength.[22,24,25] Patients should be evaluated for delirium at least once per shift during periods of greatest wakefulness (eg, after a spontaneous awakening trial).[22]

A patient's risk for delirium depends on a complex interplay between predisposing and precipitating risk factors. Although more than 100 different ICU delirium risk factors have been reported, only 18 putative, nondrug risk factors for delirium are supported by either a strong or moderate level of evidence (**Table 1**).[26] Outside of an older age itself, a history of cognitive impairment, living alone, and hypertension are particularly common

Table 1
Nonmedication risk factors for delirium

	Strong Risk Factors	Moderate Risk Factors
Nonmodifiable	• Older age • History of dementia • Pre-ICU emergency surgery or trauma • Higher severity of illness • Need for mechanical ventilation • Sepsis • Metabolic acidosis	• Living alone (elderly) • Alcohol consumption • Hypertension • Moderate cognitive impairment • Admission with infection or respiratory insufficiency • Medical admission
Modifiable	• Iatrogenic coma • Restraint use • Patient immobility	• Excessive ambient noise • Admission to an ICU room lacking features to help maintain orientation and circadian normalcy

in older adults. An important link exists between sleep disruption and delirium.[27] Cognitive dysfunction may occur during periods of severe sleep deficit, cerebral perfusion and cortical metabolism are altered during delirium and altered sleep states, and altered circadian rhythmicity may influence the fluctuation of delirium symptoms.[28]

Treatment options for delirium in the ICU remain limited.[29] Therefore, clinicians should focus their efforts on delirium prevention and risk-reduction strategies.[22,30] All predisposing (eg, older age) and some precipitating (eg, severity of illness) delirium risk factors are not reversible. However, such precipitating factors as patient immobility, application of patient restraints, excessive ambient noise, and admission to an ICU room without windows, clocks, or other features conducive to the maintenance of orientation and circadian normalcy are usually modifiable and important for clinicians to consider.[22,26]

POLYPHARMACY AS A RISK FACTOR FOR DELIRIUM

Several medications used in the critically ill have been associated with delirium[31] (Table 2). The number of medications administered in the ICU setting is large, end-organ dysfunction may influence drug response, sepsis or stroke may impair blood-brain barrier integrity, and medications with psychoactive properties can mimic delirium.[32] Although many of the proposed pathways for drug-induced delirium overlap with those for delirium itself (eg, anticholinergic activity, GABAminergic activity) few are confirmed.[32] Home medications, such as benzodiazepines or opioids that are stopped at the time of ICU admission, may cause a withdrawal syndrome the symptoms of which are similar to delirium.

Ascribing delirium at the ICU bedside solely to the use of a particular medication, however, is fraught with potential limitations.[33] The causes for delirium in the ICU are usually multifactorial and seldom obvious, the temporal relationship between medication initiation and delirium onset remains poorly characterized, and medications (eg, benzodiazepines) that may be used to treat delirium-associated agitation may also influence delirium recognition and its duration.[34]

The ICU drug-associated delirium literature consists primarily of case series and uncontrolled cohort studies, rather than cohort studies that incorporate time-dependent multivariable models or randomized controlled trials.[33] Therefore, for most medications attributed to delirium causality remains unclear. With medication exposure, most other delirium risk factors, and the presence of delirium itself often varying

Table 2
ICU medications commonly associated with delirium

Category of Medication	Examples	Mechanism
Analgesics	Fentanyl	GABA antagonism
	Hydromorphone	GABA antagonism
	Morphine	GABA antagonism
	NSAIDs	Anticholinergic activity
Anti-infectives	Acyclovir	Unknown
	Amphotericin	Unknown
	Cefepime	GABA antagonism
	Linezolid	Serotonergic dysfunction
	Macrolides	Unknown
	Quinolones	GABA antagonism
	Voriconazole	Unknown
Anticholinergics	Atropine	Anticholinergic activity
	Benztropine	Anticholinergic activity
Anticonvulsants	Levetiracetam	Unknown
Antidepressants	SSRIs	Serotonergic dysfunction
Antihistamines	Diphenhydramine	Anticholinergic activity
Cardiac medications	α-Blockers	Anticholinergic activity
	Amiodarone	Anticholinergic activity
Antipsychotics	Haloperidol	Anticholinergic activity
	Olanzapine	Anticholinergic activity
Corticosteroids	Dexamethasone	Glucocorticoid activity
	Hydrocortisone	Glucocorticoid activity
	Methylprednisolone	Glucocorticoid activity
Dopaminergics	Amantadine	Excess dopaminergic activity
	Bromocriptine	Excess dopaminergic activity
Prokinetics	Metoclopramide	Excess glucocorticoid activity
Sedatives	Ketamine	NMDA antagonism
	Lorazepam	GABA antagonism
	Midazolam	GABA antagonism
	Propofol	GABA antagonism

Abbreviations: GABA, γ-aminobutyric acid; NMDA, N-methyl-D-aspartate; NSAIDs, nonsteroidal anti-inflammatory drugs; SSRI, selective serotonin reuptake inhibitor.

Data from Devlin JW, Fraser GL, Riker RR. Drug-induced coma and delirium. In: Papadopoulos J, Cooper B, Kane-Gill S, et al, editors. Drug-induced complications in the critically ill patient: a guide for recognition and treatment. Chicago: Society of Critical Care Medicine; 2011. p. 107–16.

over each ICU day, sophisticated, time-dependent models are needed to evaluate the association between medication exposure and delirium occurrence.[33] An increasing number of time-dependent, multivariate analyses that incorporate Markov models to focus on the association between medication exposure (eg, benzodiazepines, corticosteroids, and anticholinergics) and the daily odds of transitioning from an awake and nondelirious state to delirium the next day have recently been published.[35–40]

A landmark 2006 study of 198 mechanically ventilated adults found that lorazepam administration was an independent risk factor for a daily transition to delirium (odds ratio [OR], 1.2; 95% confidence interval [CI], 1.1–1.4; $P = .003$).[35] A more recent analysis of 1112 critically ill adults found that midazolam administration was an independent risk factor for a daily transition to delirium (OR, 1.04; 95% CI, 1.02–1.05; $P<.001$ per every 5 mg per day of midazolam administered).[40] This latter study suggests that for every 5 mg of midazolam administered to a patient, who is awake and without delirium, there is a 4% chance that this patient will develop delirium the next ICU day. Note that this risk is additive and thus the administration of 20 mg of midazolam in a 24-hour period is associated with a 16% chance of delirium occurring the next day. The lower odds for transitioning to delirium in this latter study is a reflection of a trend over the past decade to reduce benzodiazepine dosing in an effort to promote patient wakefulness. Given that the risk for delirium-associated benzodiazepine use is dose-dependent, clinicians should use strategies known to reduce the daily amount of benzo-diazepine administered that often includes the use of a sedative associated with less delirium occurrence, such as dexmedetomidine or propofol.[22]

Despite the uncertain efficacy of corticosteroids for many critical illnesses and their extensive risk profile, corticosteroids are frequently administered in the ICU. Although corticosteroids decrease inflammation, and therefore theoretically reduce neuroin-flammation and the incidence of delirium, the results of the Dexamethasone for Cardiac Surgery trial suggest that the administration of a corticosteroid before cardiac surgery does not affect the occurrence of postoperative delirium.[41] Although delirium has long been assumed to be a potential consequence of corticosteroid use, particu-larly with high doses, its association with delirium has only recently been rigorously evaluated.[36,39]

Using multivariable Markov modeling techniques, one cohort analysis of 520 me-chanically ventilated adults with acute lung injury found that systemic corticosteroid use was significantly associated with transitioning to delirium from a nondelirious, noncomatose state.[36] However, in a larger analysis of 1112 patients, who received a corticosteroid on 35% of their ICU days at a median prednisone equivalent dose of 50 (25–75) mg, corticosteroid administration was not associated with a daily tran-sition to delirium (OR, 1.08; 95% CI, 0.89–1.32 per each 10-mg increase in predni-sone equivalent administered).[39] A secondary analysis of the 45% of patients who had severe hypoxemia (and thus likely had the acute respiratory distress syndrome) revealed a risk for delirium that remained unchanged. Differences between these two studies in the way in which additional delirium risk factors were identified and incor-porated, the daily frequency by which delirium was evaluated, and the differing pa-tient populations likely account for these discordant results. Regardless of the exact risk for delirium with corticosteroid exposure, ICU clinicians should continue to evaluate their patients daily to ensure that they are receiving the lowest effective dose.

Cholinergic deficiency has been traditionally described as an important mechanistic cause for delirium occurrence.[42] However, the few studies that have evaluated anti-cholinergic medication use and delirium occurrence in the ICU have failed to use time-dependent multinomial models or consider the effects of either increased age or the presence of an acute inflammatory state on this relationship.[43] In one prospec-tive study of 1112 critically ill adults, anticholinergic burden was calculated on a daily basis using the sum of the Anticholinergic Drug Scale score for each medication administered (median [interquartile range] = 2 [1–3]).[38] The transition from being in an "awake without delirium" state to "delirium" occurred on 562 of ICU days (6%). Us-ing a first-order Markov model that adjusted for eight covariables, a one-unit increase in the Anticholinergic Drug Scale score resulted in a nonsignificant increase in the odds of delirium occurring the next day (OR, 1.05; 95% CI, 0.99–1.10). Neither age nor the presence of acute systemic inflammation modified this relationship. Although medications without strong anticholinergic properties are preferred in the critically ill, the results of this investigation suggest that the association between anticholinergic medication use and delirium in the critically ill may not be as significant as previously thought.

POLYPHARMACY AS A SEQUELAE OF DELIRIUM TREATMENT

When delirium is identified in older adults, clinicians should focus on providing proven nonpharmacological delirium reduction strategies, such as frequent reorientation, early mobilization, and noise abatement, given their proven efficacy and low risk.[22,30] However, drugs, particularly antipsychotics and dexmedetomidine, are often initiated given the time and effort associated with implementing nonpharmacologic delirium reduction interventions coupled with the ease by which medications can be administered in the ICU setting. Antipsychotics are given off label to more than 10% of ICU patients, and often at high and excessive doses.[44–46] Continuation of newly initiated antipsychotics beyond the care setting and context for which they were prescribed is frequent.[44,47] Moreover, patients with delirium who are agitated may also be initiated on benzodiazepines; opioids; or sedating anticonvulsants, such as phenobarbital.[48] These factors make delirium an important contributor to polypharmacy in critically ill older adults.

The initiation of antipsychotic medication in hospitalized patients has raised concern. Extended posthospital antipsychotic use may be associated with serious safety concerns[49,50]; in older adults with dementia, this use may increase short-term mortality.[51] The 2015 Beers criteria advocate that antipsychotics be avoided in all delirious patients.[11] Recently the Centers for Medicare and Medicaid Services have proposed that antipsychotic use in hospitalized older adults, including the critically ill, should be restricted to only those patients where the patient is threatening harm to themselves or others.[52]

Although it is clear that antipsychotics and other medications, such as dexmedetomidine, may sometimes be inappropriately initiated in older adults with delirium in the ICU, there are important considerations that support the use of these agents in some circumstances. To date, eight prospective, randomized studies have evaluated various drugs to treat delirium in critically ill patients (**Table 3**).[53–60] Among the studies evaluating antipsychotics, none incorporated a formal delirium risk factor reduction protocol,[61] antipsychotic dosing regimens were not based on formal pharmacokinetic and pharmacodynamic evaluations,[62] and none considered pharmacogenomic variability.[63] Large, multicenter antipsychotic delirium prevention[64] and treatment trials[65] are nearing completion. Until the results of these studies are available, the routine role for antipsychotics in critically ill older adults remains inconclusive.

Antipsychotics have been administered for decades to reduce agitation, to treat fear or its potentially violent manifestation, and to help promote sleep. Decade-old recommendations to treat delirium with haloperidol, and more recently quetiapine, can be found in practice guidelines[22,66] and textbooks.[67] Although use of antipsychotics in the ICU is currently not supported by rigorous evidence,[68] studies to support pharmacologic alternatives to antipsychotics in the ICU, other than dexmedetomidine, are nonexistent and antipsychotics may reduce potentially deliriogenic interventions, such as restraints.[22,29]

A short course of antipsychotics may be indicated to treat agitation, particularly in patients for whom respiratory depression is of concern. Recent studies demonstrate the benefit of low-dose haloperidol in reducing agitation in patients with delirium[59] or subsyndromal delirium.[69] The fact that dexmedetomidine, an alternative to haloperidol in patients with delirium who are severely agitated, is associated with bradycardia and hypotension, a high acquisition cost and a requirement it be administered as a continuous infusion in a monitored setting, often precludes its administration.[60] Lastly, there may be a role for antipsychotics at night in patients who report insomnia, in whom nonpharmacologic sleep improvement interventions fail, because sleep architecture (an important determinant of outcome) is less disrupted with antipsychotics than with benzodiazepines or propofol.[70,71]

Table 3
Randomized studies evaluating an antipsychotic or dexmedetomidine delirium treatment strategy in the critically ill

Author, Year	Skrobik et al,[53] 2004	Pandharipande et al,[54] 2007	Ruokonen et al,[55] 2009	Riker et al,[56] 2009	Devlin et al,[58] 2010	Girard et al,[57] 2010	Page et al,[59] 2013	Reade et al,[60] 2016
Baseline delirium (%)	100	61	NR	60	100	49	NR	100
Patient population (%)	Surgical = 95 Intubated = 0	Medical = 70 Intubated = 100	Medical = 53 Intubated = 100	Medical = 86 Intubated = 100	Medical = 75 Intubated = 81	Medical = 62 Intubated = 100	Medical = 65 Intubated = 100	Medical = 41 Intubated = 100
Intervention	Olanzapine, 5 mg PO/ENT daily (n = 28)	Dexmed, up to 1.5 μg/kg/h IV (n = 52)	Dexmed, up to 1.4 μg/kg/h IV (n = 41)	Dexmed, up to 1.4 μg/kg/h IV (n = 244)	Quetiapine, up to 200 mg PO/ENT q 12 h (n = 18)	Ziprasidone, 40 mg PO/ENT up to q 6 h (n = 30)	Haloperidol, 2.5 mg IV q 8 h (n = 71)	Dexmed, up to 1.5 μg/kg/h IV (n = 39)
Control	Haloperidol, 2.5–5 mg PO/ENT q 8 h (n = 45)	Lorazepam, up to 10 mg/h (n = 51)	Midazolam, up to 0.2 mg/kg/h or propofol, up to 66 μg/kg/min (n = 44)	Midazolam, up to 0.1 mg/kg/h (n = 122)	Placebo PO/ENT (n = 18)	C1: haloperidol, 5 mg PO/ENT q 6 h (n = 35) C2: placebo IM/PO/ENT (n = 36)	Placebo IV (n = 70)	Placebo IV (n = 32)
Delirium present at end of study period (%)	NR	79 vs 82; P = .65	44 vs 25; P = .035	54 vs 77; P<.001	NR	69 vs 77; P = .28	NR	NR
Duration of delirium	NR	Delirium-free days 9 (5–11) vs 7 (5–11); P = .09	NR	NR	36 (12–87) vs 120 (60–195) h; P = .006	4 (2–7) vs 4 (2–8) (C1) vs 2 (0–5) (C2) d; P = .93	5 (2–8) vs 5 (1–8) d; P = .53	Time to resolution 23 (13–54) vs 40 (25–76) h; P = .01

Data presented as median (interquartile range).
Abbreviations: Dexmed, dexmedetomidine; ENT, enterally; IM, intramuscular; IV, intravenous; NR, not reported; PO, by mouth; q, every.
Data from Refs.[53–60]

STRATEGIES TO REDUCE THE POLYPHARMACY-DELIRIUM CYCLE

Quality improvement efforts that mandate delirium screening efforts in the ICU are critical to reduce drug-associated delirium in this setting.[22] The diagnosis of drug-induced delirium is challenging and is generally one of exclusion based on the appearance (and resolution) of delirium relative to medication use.[26,32] Given that risk factors for ICU delirium are often modifiable, a careful pre-emptive evaluation of environmental- and medication-related risk factors associated with delirium should be conducted before pharmacologic delirium treatment interventions are considered.[23,26,32]

The medication profile for all ICU patients should be reviewed daily. Redundant drugs should be discontinued and for all required medications should be administered at their lowest effective dose.[11] In patients with delirium, medications known to cause delirium should be stopped and alternative medications initiated. If the use of an at-risk medication cannot be avoided, the lowest dose of the medication should be prescribed and the duration of therapy should be as short as possible.[70] Common strategies used to reduce medication-associated delirium are presented in **Box 1**. Removal or reduction of delirium risk factors is the most important strategy when resolving delirium symptoms and limiting associated sequelae.[23,29,30] Mnemonics, such as "I-C-U-D-E-L-I-R-I-U-M-S," are used by clinicians to help remember the common risk factors and causes for delirium in the ICU when evaluating a patient who has developed delirium in to identify potentially reversible causes[72] (**Table 4**).

Professional organizations and their members, such as the Society of Critical Care Medicine, devote substantial resources and efforts to develop high-quality clinical practice guidelines and quality improvement efforts.[23,73,74] These guidelines and other expert panels have identified important gaps in knowledge surrounding the role of antipsychotics in ICU practice, furthering the research agenda in this area.[23,75]

Critical care pharmacists play an important role in reducing polypharmacy, preventing drug-associated delirium and making recommendations regarding its appropriate treatment (**Box 2**).[75] Medication reconciliation should be a mandatory at time of the ICU admission and discharge and should involve nurses, pharmacists, and

---

Box 1
Factors associated with polypharmacy and adverse drug events in critically ill older adults

- Failure to account for age- and critical care–related pharmacokinetic changes
- Failure to avoid high-risk drugs whenever possible
- Failure to screen for pain, sedation, and delirium
- Initiation of a new medication to treat a side effect from another
- Failure to regularly down-titrate or discontinue medications
- Failure to recognize drug-associated adverse effects
- Reinitiation of a medication a patient had stopped taking before the ICU admission
- Failure to consider pre-ICU over-the-counter medication, herbal, alcohol, or recreational drug use
- Failure to consider risks of reactions from medication withdrawal
- Lack of involvement of a critical care pharmacist in daily ICU care
- Lack of involvement of family and friends in daily ICU care
- Lack of medication reconciliation at the time of ICU discharge

Table 4
Mnemonic for risk factors and causes of ICU delirium: "ICU DELIRIUM (S)"

*I*atrogenic exposure	Diagnostic procedures, therapeutic interventions, or a harmful occurrence deemed not to be a natural consequence of the patient's illness
*C*ognitive impairment	Pre-existing dementia, stroke, or depression
*U*se of restraints and catheters	Avoid use of restraints and bladder catheters unless clinically indicated
*D*rugs	Sedatives (eg, benzodiazepines) and medications with anticholinergic activity Abrupt cessation of smoking or alcohol Withdrawal from chronic sedative use
*E*lderly	Patients older than 65 y
*L*aboratory abnormalities	Hyponatremia, azotemia, hyperbilirubinemia, hypocalcemia, metabolic acidosis
*I*nfection	Sepsis and severe sepsis Urinary or respiratory tract infections
*R*espiratory	Respiratory failure (P_{CO_2} >45 mm Hg or P_{O_2} <55 mm Hg or oxygen saturation <88%) COPD, ARDS, PE
*I*ntracranial perfusion	Presence of hypertension, hypotension, hemorrhage, stroke, or tumor
*U*rinary/fecal retention	Urinary retention or fecal impaction, especially in elderly and postoperative patients
*M*yocardial	Myocardial causes including myocardial infarction, acute heart failure, or arrhythmia
*S*leep and *S*ensory deprivation	Alterations of the sleep cycle and sleep deprivation Nonavailability of glasses or hearing devices

Abbreviations: ARDS, acute respiratory distress syndrome; COPD, chronic obstructive pulmonary disease; PE, pulmonary embolus.
Courtesy of Wes Ely, MD, Nashville, TN; with permission.

Box 2
Strategies to reduce medication-related delirium in the ICU

- Avoid polypharmacy and ensure that all medications are dosed appropriately
- Consider medication withdrawal effects (particularly benzodiazepines)
- Avoid anticholinergic medications when possible
- Avoid benzodiazepines when possible (including use as a sleep aid)
- Avoid use of nonbenzodiazepine sleep aids when possible
- Use the lowest effective corticosteroid dose
- Use the lowest effective opioid dose to control pain/optimize nonopioid analgesic
- Avoid metoclopramide when possible
- If delirium occurs with levetiracetam consider other anticonvulsant options
- Reassess need for continued antibiotic therapy
- Monitor diuretic therapy for signs of dehydration and/or electrolyte abnormalities

Data from Devlin JW, Fraser GL, Riker RR. Drug-induced coma and delirium. In: Papadopoulos J, Cooper B, Kane-Gill S, et al, editors. Drug-induced complications in the critically ill patient: a guide for recognition and treatment. Chicago: Society of Critical Care Medicine; 2011. p. 107–16.

physicians.[76,77] Family members can play a useful role in identifying the medications that patients were taking at the time of admission.

SUMMARY

Polypharmacy is a common sequelae of ICU admission and is associated with increased medication-associated adverse events, drug interactions, and health care costs. Delirium is prevalent in critically ill geriatric patients and medications, many of which are commonly administered in the ICU, remain an underappreciated modifiable risk for delirium in this population. Pharmacologic ICU delirium treatment interventions, particularly antipsychotics, may contribute to polypharmacy during and after the ICU stay. Critically ill patients should be regularly screened for delirium with a validated instrument; all assessment results should be discussed during bedside rounds. The medication list for a patient with delirium should be carefully reviewed and medications known to be associated with delirium should be discontinued or replaced with medications not known to increase delirium risk. Nonpharmacologic interventions, such as early mobilization, environmental modulation, and sleep protocols, should be optimized before pharmacologic options are used in a patient with delirium given their far-stronger evidence profile. Pain should be considered and treated in a patient with delirium who is agitated before antipsychotic or dexmedetomidine therapy is initiated. Current evidence does not support the routine use of antipsychotics in older adults with delirium. Critical care pharmacists and formal medication reconciliation efforts are important strategies to reduce polypharmacy including the post-ICU use of antipsychotics in older adults who continue to have delirium.

REFERENCES

1. Fowler RA, Adhikari NK, Bhagwanjee S. Clinical review: critical care in the global context–disparities in burden of illness, access, and economics. Crit Care 2008; 12(5):225.
2. Fuchs L, Chronaki CE, Park S, et al. ICU admission characteristics and mortality rates among elderly and very elderly patients. Intensive Care Med 2012;38(10): 1654–61.
3. Balas MC, Devlin JW, Verceles AC, et al. Adapting the ABCDEF bundle to meet the needs of patients requiring prolonged mechanical ventilation in the long-term acute care hospital setting: historical perspectives and practical implications. Semin Respir Crit Care Med 2016;37(1):119–35.
4. Bell CM, Brener SS, Gunraj N, et al. Association of ICU or hospital admission with unintentional discontinuation of medications for chronic diseases. JAMA 2011; 306:840–7.
5. Budnitz DS, Pollock DA, Weidenbach KN, et al. National surveillance of emergency department visits for outpatient adverse drug events. JAMA 2006; 296(15):1858–66.
6. Jolivot PA, Hindlet P, Pichereau C, et al. A systematic review of adult admissions to ICUs related to adverse drug events. Crit Care 2014;18(6):643.
7. Qato DM, Wilder J, Schumm LP, et al. Changes in prescription and over-the-counter medication and dietary supplement use among older adults in the United States, 2005 vs 2011. JAMA Intern Med 2016;176(4):473–82.
8. Cullen DJ, Sweitzer BJ, Bates DW, et al. Preventable adverse drug events in hospitalized patients: a comparative study of intensive care and general care units. Crit Care Med 1997;25:1289–97.

9. Devlin JW, Barletta JF. Principles of drug dosing in the critically ill. In: Parillo JW, Dellinger RP, editors. Critical care medicine: principles of diagnosis and management in the adult. 3rd edition. Philadelphia: Mosby-Elsevier; 2008. p. 343–76.

10. Lat I, Micek S, Janzen J, et al. Off-label medication use in adult critical care patients. J Crit Care 2011;26:89–94.

11. By the American Geriatrics Society 2015 Beers Criteria Update Expert Panel. American Geriatrics Society 2015 updated Beers criteria for potentially inappropriate medication use in older adults. J Am Geriatr Soc 2015;63:2227–46.

12. Morandi A, Vasilevskis EE, Pandharipande PP, et al. Inappropriate medications in elderly ICU survivors: where to intervene? Arch Intern Med 2011;171(11):1032–4.

13. Floroff CK, Slattum PW, Harpe SE, et al. Potentially inappropriate medication use is associated with clinical outcomes in critically ill elderly patients with neurological injury. Neurocrit Care 2014;21(3):526–33.

14. Morandi A, Vasilevskis E, Pandharipande PP, et al. Inappropriate medication prescriptions in elderly adults surviving an intensive care unit hospitalizations. J Am Geriatr Soc 2013;61:1128–34.

15. Cook RI, Render M, Woods DD. Gaps in the continuity of care and progress on patient safety. BMJ 2000;320:7910794.

16. Scales DC, Fisher HD, Li P, et al. Unintentional continuation of medications intended for acute illness after hospital discharge: a population-based cohort study. J Gen Intern Med 2015;31:196–202.

17. American Psychiatric Association. Diagnostic and statistical manual of mental disorders: DSM-IV. 4th edition. Washington, DC: American Psychiatric Association; 1994.

18. Marquis F, Ouimet S, Riker R, et al. Individual delirium symptoms: do they matter? Crit Care Med 2007;35:2533–7.

19. Ely EW, Shintani A, Truman B, et al. Delirium as a predictor of mortality in mechanically ventilated patients in the intensive care unit. JAMA 2004;291:1753–62.

20. Salluh JI, Wang H, Scheider EB, et al. Outcome of delirium in critically ill patients: systematic review and meta-analysis. BMJ 2015;350:h2538.

21. Pandharipande PP, Girard TD, Jackson JC, et al. Long-term cognitive impairment after critical illness. BRAIN-ICU Study Investigators. N Engl J Med 2013;369:1306–16.

22. Barr J, Fraser GL, Puntillo K, et al. Clinical practice guidelines for the management of pain, agitation and delirium in adult ICU patients. Crit Care Med 2013;41(1):263–306.

23. Devlin JW, Fong JJ, Fraser GL, et al. Delirium assessment in the critically ill. Intensive Care Med 2007;33:929–40.

24. Ely EW, Inouye SK, Bernard GR, et al. Delirium in mechanically ventilated patients: validity and reliability of the confusion assessment method for the intensive care unit (CAM-ICU). JAMA 2001;286:2703–10.

25. Bergeron N, Dubois MJ, Dumont M, et al. Intensive care delirium screening checklist: evaluation of a new screening tool. Intensive Care Med 2001;27:859–64.

26. Zaal IJ, Devlin JW, Peelen LM, et al. A systematic review of risk factors for delirium in the ICU. Crit Care Med 2015;43:40–7.

27. Pisani MA, Friese RS, Gehlbach BK, et al. Sleep in the intensive care unit. Am J Respir Crit Care Med 2015;191:731–8.

28. Oldman MA, Lee HB, Desan PH. Circadian rhythm disruption in the critically ill: an opportunity for improving outcomes. Crit Care Med 2016;44:207–17.

29. Serafim RB, Bozza FA, Soares M, et al. Pharmacologic prevention and treatment of delirium in intensive care patients: a systematic review. J Crit Care 2015;30: 799–807.

30. Trogrlić Z, van der Jagt M, Bakker J, et al. A systematic review of implementation strategies for assessment, prevention, and management of ICU delirium and their effect on clinical outcomes. Crit Care 2015;19:157.

31. Available at: www.Micromedex.com. Accessed May 28, 2016.

32. Devlin JW, Fraser GL, Riker RR. Drug-induced coma and delirium. In: Papadopoulos J, Cooper B, Kane-Gill S, et al, editors. Drug-induced complications in the critically ill patient: a guide for recognition and treatment. 1st edition. Chicago: Society of Critical Care Medicine; 2011. p. 164–81.

33. Devlin JW, Zaal IJ, Slooter AJ. Clarifying the confusion surrounding drug-associated delirium in the ICU. Crit Care Med 2014;42:1565–6.

34. Patel SB, Poston JT, Pohlman A, et al. Rapidly reversible, sedation-related delirium versus persistent delirium in the intensive care unit. Am J Respir Crit Care Med 2014;189:658–65.

35. Pandharipande P, Shintani A, Peterson J, et al. Lorazepam is an independent risk factor for transitioning to delirium in intensive care unit patients. Anesthesiology 2006;104(1):21–6.

36. Schreiber MP, Colantuoni E, Bienvenu OJ, et al. Corticosteroids and transition to delirium in patients with acute lung injury. Crit Care Med 2014;42(6):1480–6.

37. Kamdar BB, Niessen T, Colantuoni E, et al. Delirium transitions in the medical ICU: exploring the role of sleep quality and other factors. Crit Care Med 2015; 43:135–41.

38. Wolters AE, Zaal IJ, Veldhuijzen DS, et al. Anticholinergic medication use and transition to delirium in critically ill patients: a prospective cohort study. Crit Care Med 2015;43(9):1846–52.

39. Wolters AE, Veldhuijzzen DS, Zaal IJ, et al. Systemic corticosteroids and transition to delirium in critically ill patients. Crit Care Med 2015;43(12):e585–8.

40. Zaal IJ, Devlin JW, Hazelbag M, et al. Benzodiazepine-associated delirium in critically ill adults. Intensive Care Med 2015;41:2130–7.

41. Sauër AM, Slooter AJC, Veldhuijzen DS, et al. Intraoperative dexamethasone and delirium after cardiac surgery: a randomized clinical trial. Anesth Analg 2014; 119(5):1046–52.

42. Hshieh TT, Fong TG, Marcantonio ER, et al. Cholinergic deficiency hypothesis in delirium: a synthesis of current evidence. J Gerontol A Biol Sci Med Sci 2008;63: 764–72.

43. Tune L, Carr S, Cooper T, et al. Association of anticholinergic activity of prescribed medications with postoperative delirium. J Neuropsychiatry Clin Neurosci 1993;5:208–10.

44. Marshall J, Herzig SJ, Howell MD, et al. Antipsychotic utilization in the intensive care unit and in transitions of care. J Crit Care 2016;33:119–24.

45. Swan JT, Fitousis K, Hall JB, et al. Antipsychotic use and diagnosis of delirium in the intensive care unit. Crit Care 2012;16:R84.

46. Herzig SJ, Rothwerg MB, Guess JR, et al. Antipsychotic medication utilization in nonpsychiatric hospitalizations. J Hosp Med 2016;11:543–9.

47. Rowe AS, Hamilton LA, Curtis RA, et al. Risk factors for discharge on new antipsychotic medication after admission to an intensive care unit. J Crit Care 2015;30:1283–6.

48. Devlin JW, Bhat S, Roberts RJ, et al. Current perceptions and practices surrounding the recognition and treatment of delirium in the intensive care unit: a survey of

250 critical care pharmacists from eight states. Ann Pharmacother 2011;45: 1217–29.

49. Hwang YJ, Dixon SN, Reiss JP, et al. Atypical antipsychotic drugs and the risk for acute kidney injury and other adverse outcomes in older adults: a population-based cohort study. Ann Intern Med 2014;161:242–8.

50. Trifirò G, Gambassi G, Sen EF, et al. Association of community acquired pneumonia with antipsychotic drug use in elderly patients: a nested case-control study. Ann Intern Med 2010;152:418–25.

51. Wang PS, Schneeweiss S, Avorn J, et al. Risk of death in elderly users of conventional vs. atypical antipsychotic medications. N Engl J Med 2005;353:2335–41.

52. Use of antipsychotics in older adults in the inpatient hospital setting. Available at: https://www.cms.gov/Medicare/Quality-Initiatives-Patient-Assessment-Instruments/MMS/CallforPublicComment.html#28. Accessed May 28, 2016.

53. Skrobik YK, Bergeron N, Dumont M, et al. Olanzapine vs haloperidol: treating delirium in a critical care setting. Intensive Care Med 2004;30:444–9.

54. Pandharipande PP, Pun BT, Herr DL, et al. Effect of sedation with dexmedetomidine vs lorazepam on acute brain dysfunction in mechanically ventilated patients: the MENDS randomized controlled trial. JAMA 2007;298:2644–53.

55. Ruokonen E, Parviainen I, Jakob S, et al. Dexmedetomidine versus propofol/midazolam for long-term sedation during mechanical ventilation. Intensive Care Med 2009;35:282–90.

56. Riker RR, Shehabi Y, Bokesch PM, et al. Dexmedetomidine vs midazolam for sedation of critically ill patients: a randomized trial. JAMA 2009;301:489–99.

57. Girard TD, Pandharipande PP, Carson SS, et al. Feasibility, efficacy, and safety of antipsychotics for intensive care unit delirium: the MIND randomized, placebo-controlled trial. Crit Care Med 2010;38:428–37.

58. Devlin JW, Roberts RJ, Fong JJ, et al. Efficacy and safety of quetiapine in critically ill patients with delirium: a prospective, multicenter, randomized, double-blind, placebo-controlled pilot study. Crit Care Med 2010;38:419–27.

59. Page VJ, Ely EW, Gates S, et al. Effect of intravenous haloperidol on the duration of delirium and coma in critically ill patients (Hope-ICU): a randomised, double-blind, placebo-controlled trial. Lancet Respir Med 2013;1:515–23.

60. Reade MC, Eastwood GM, Bellomo R, et al. Effect of dexmedetomidine added to standard care on ventilator-free time in patients with agitated delirium: a randomized clinical trial. JAMA 2016;315:1460–8.

61. Balas MC, Vasilevskis EE, Olsen KM, et al. Effectiveness and safety of the awakening and breathing coordination, delirium monitoring/management, and early exercise/mobility bundle. Crit Care Med 2014;42:1024–36.

62. Smith BS, Yogaratnam D, Levasseur-Franklin KE, et al. Introduction to drug pharmacokinetics in the critically ill patient. Chest 2012;141:1327–36.

63. Devlin JW, Skrobik Y. Antipsychotics for the prevention and treatment of delirium in the intensive care unit: what is their role? Harv Rev Psychiatry 2011;19:59–67.

64. van den Boogaard M, Slooter AJ, Brüggemann RJ, et al. Prevention of ICU delirium and delirium-related outcome with haloperidol: a study protocol for a multicenter randomized controlled trial. Trials 2013;14:400.

65. The modifying the impact of ICU-associated neurological dysfunction USA (MIND-USA) study. Available at: https://clinicaltrials.gov/ct2/show/NCT0121 1522?term=MIND+USA&rank. Accessed May 28, 2016.

66. American Psychiatric Association. Practice guideline for the treatment of patients with delirium. Am J Psychiatry 1999;156:1–20.

67. Caplan JP. Diagnosis and treatment of agitation and delirium in the intensive care unit patient. In: Irwin RS, Rippe JM, editors. Irwin and Rippe's intensive care medicine. 7th edition. Philadelphia: Lippincott, William & Wilkins; 2012. p. 2073–9.

68. Neufeld KM, Yue J, Robinson TN, et al. Antipsychotic medication for prevention and treatment of delirium in hospitalized patients: a systematic review and meta-analysis. J Am Geratr Soc 2016;64:705–14.

69. Al-Qadheeb NS, Skrobik Y, Schumaker G, et al. Preventing ICU subsyndromal delirium conversion to delirium with low-dose IV haloperidol: a double-blind, placebo-controlled, pilot study. Crit Care Med 2016;44:583–91.

70. Kondili E, Alexopoulou C, Xirouchaki N, et al. Effects of propofol on sleep quality in mechanically ventilated critically ill patients: a physiological study. Intensive Care Med 2012;38:1640–6.

71. Oto J, Yamamoto K, Koike S, et al. Effect of daily sedative interruption on sleep stages of mechanically ventilated patients receiving midazolam by infusion. Anaesth Intensive Care 2011;39:392–400.

72. Availabe at: www.ICUdelirium.org. Accessed May 28, 2016.

73. Society of Critical Care Medicine ICU Liberation Campaign. Available at: http://www.iculiberation.org. Accessed May 28, 2016.

74. AGS/NIA Delirium Conference Writing Group, Planning Committee and Faculty. The American Geriatrics Society/National Institute on Aging Bedside-to-Benchmark Conference: research agenda on delirium in older adults. J Am Geriatr Soc 2015; 63:843–52.

75. Preslaski CR, Lat I, MacLaren R, et al. Pharmacist contributions as members of the multidisciplinary ICU team. Chest 2013;144(5):1687–95.

76. Varkey P, Cunningham J, O'Meara J, et al. Multidisciplinary approach to inpatient medication reconciliation in an academic setting. Am J Health Syst Pharm 2007; 64:850–4.

77. Rodehover C, Fearing D. Medication reconciliation in acute care: ensuring an accurate drug regimen on admission and discharge. Jt Comm J Qual Patient Saf 2005;31:406–13.

Geriatric Polypharmacy

Pharmacist as Key Facilitator in Assessing for Falls Risk

Michelle A. Fritsch, PharmD[a],*, Penny S. Shelton, PharmD[b]

KEYWORDS

• Falls • Medication • Pharmacist • Geriatric • Falls assessment • Patient safety

KEY POINTS

- The health care burden associated with the growing incidence of falls among the elderly is anticipated to worsen.
- Pharmacists are members of the patient health care team not commonly thought of but uniquely positioned to help assess and address falls risk.
- Patients with positive falls screenings should be comprehensively assessed to identify and address multiple causative factors associated with falls.
- A 6-step, comprehensive falls assessment including falls-associated drugs and medical conditions is described, including implementation concepts based on pharmacy practice setting.

INTRODUCTION

Each year millions of falls-related injuries occur among individuals age 65 or older. As many as 1 in 3 older adults fall annually, and the toll from these falls generates a significant public health problem in the United States.[1] Falls often result in injuries, which require emergent care (2.5 million annually) and hospitalization (700,000 annually).[2] Falls-related injuries and subsequent debilitation can result in short- or long-term loss of independence.[3] Most tragically, despite much attention being focused on falls awareness, the falls death rate among older adults has continued to increase annually over the past decade, with an increase of approximately 7100 deaths between 2005 and 2011.[4] The Centers for Disease Control and Prevention (CDC) reported an adjusted direct medical cost for falls in 2013 as totaling $34 billion.[5,6] Because of the aging of our society, if significant proactive interventions are not put in place,

[a] Meds MASH, LLC, 16326 Matthews Road, Monkton, MD 21111, USA; [b] North Carolina Association of Pharmacists, 1101 Slater Road, Suite 110, Durham, NC 27703, USA
* Corresponding author.
E-mail address: michelle@medsmash.com

Clin Geriatr Med 33 (2017) 205–223
http://dx.doi.org/10.1016/j.cger.2017.01.003
0749-0690/17/© 2017 Elsevier Inc. All rights reserved.

geriatric.theclinics.com

both the number of and the costs to treat falls injuries are anticipated to continue to increase.

There are numerous factors proven to be associated with increased falls risk among the elderly. Medications are often implicated. Therefore, pharmacists can be instrumental in assessing and reducing falls risk. Falls and falls risk are particularly elevated during transitions of care, and pharmacists in both outpatient and inpatient settings have the ability to provide falls-risk reducing services.[7,8] Pharmacists' intensive education and training in medication therapy management are greatly needed to help improve patient safety.

In the outpatient setting, although commonplace for patients to see more than one physician or prescriber for their care, patients have been strongly encouraged to use one pharmacy. Using one pharmacy allows the pharmacist, after obtaining additional information regarding over-the-counter (OTC) medicines, herbal supplements, and illicit or recreational substances to review the entire medication regimen and identify actual or potential medication-related problems. This type of comprehensive medication therapy review can be conducted as part of an overall falls risk assessment and tailored to identify and address the use of falls risk-inducing drugs (FRIDs).

Pharmacists can do more than just identify falls risk. Casteel and colleagues[9] found pharmacists' recommendations for safer alternatives to reduce falls risk without compromising achievement of desired therapeutic goals. Another recent pilot program demonstrated the value of falls risk assessment within a community pharmacy setting, where identification of known FRIDs followed by medication change or dose-lowering recommendations resulted in a significant decrease in the use of FRIDs.[10]

A well-conducted, pharmacist-provided falls assessment and intervention can make a difference; however, it is the opinion of the authors that in order to substantially improve the public health concerns associated with falls among the elderly, an interprofessional approach to the problem is required. Given that medications are frequently a culprit, pharmacists, regardless of practice setting, must proactively address falls risk as part of that interprofessional team, and the information gleaned from their falls-based assessment will frequently necessitate triage and patient referral for those who need further assessment and falls risk-reducing services (**Box 1**).

Box 1
The pharmacist as an interprofessional falls-risk reducing team member

The following are examples of frequent professionals to whom pharmacists may need to refer patients based on the falls assessment findings:

    Physicians (eg, general practitioner, geriatrician, neurologist, endocrinologist, podiatrist)
        For appropriate workup of medical conditions as identified elsewhere in this publication
    Physical therapist
        For strengthening and gait improvement
    Occupational therapist
        For improvement in activities of daily living and in-home functioning and safety assessment
        For assessing patient for appropriate falls risk reduction aids
    Home improvement handyman/contractor
        For assessment, building or renovating changes to reduce in-home falls hazards (assure contractor is licensed and insured and a certified aging-in-place specialist)

Falls happen in all settings and the morbidity and mortality, as well as direct and in-direct costs associated with falls, have spurred the development of falls-related quality indicators in the care of patients. The Agency for Healthcare Research and Quality has called for improvement in the patient safety culture within hospitals, and the Center for Medicare and Medicaid's star ratings and quality measures on falls have elevated the importance of falls prevention among institutional settings, where inpatient and consul-tant pharmacists have become a vital resource for reducing falls and falls risk. The com-munity pharmacist has long been acknowledged as the most accessible health care provider, which uniquely positions the pharmacist as the member of the health care team who can use their frequent interaction with patients to observe, assess, intervene, and monitor FRIDs as well as other falls risk factors. Today, most seniors live indepen-dently or with family members in the community; as previously noted, falling is highly prevalent among this population. However, less than half of patients who fall speak to their health care providers about falling[11]; therefore, it is critically important for phar-macists to proactively ask about and assess their patients for falls.

TOOLS FOR FALLS ASSESSMENT

There are several tools that have been developed and used to identify patients at risk for falls and to minimize those risks. A tool with objective measures, quantifiable scoring, and quick administration is preferred for an initial assessment. Many institu-tions and outpatient practices use tools to screen for falls risks. Patients identified to be at risk can then be assessed with a more in-depth tool to identify specific modifi-able risk factors.

The Agency for Healthcare Research and Quality has made available an in-depth toolkit to assist hospitals with falls reduction. This multisystem toolkit is comprehen-sive and engages many practitioners within the hospital setting. It lacks specificity with FRIDs and risk-increasing medical conditions.[12] Similarly, the Johns Hopkins Falls Risk Assessment Tool is commonly used by nurses in the acute care setting due to ease of administration, but the tool lacks specificity for FRIDs and medical conditions.[13]

The CDC published the Stopping Elderly Accidents, Deaths, and Injuries (STEADI) Toolkit in 2015.[14] STEADI has been piloted within electronic medical record systems such as Epic and GE Centricity[15] and is proposed as a regular component of Medicare Annual Wellness Visits (MAWV) in the National Council on Aging Falls Free 2015 initia-tive.[16] In the STEADI toolkit, falls risk is addressed in an algorithmic fashion that des-ignates the depth of assessment based on identified risks. The toolkit highlights the importance of certain commonly associated FRIDs without guidance for medication and medical condition screening and intervention. The sections addressing FRIDs and falls-associated medical conditions are limited to the most commonly associated with falls.

Furthermore, practitioners across the country use a variety of approaches to falls risk assessment. Both a lack of standardization and limited comprehensive elements within existing screening tools reduce the effectiveness of these screenings for indi-vidual patients.

In the fall of 2016, the American Society of Consultant Pharmacists and the National Council on Aging launched a tool intended to be a companion and enhancement to STEADI (Cameron K and colleagues, Companion guide reference from fall 2016, un-published data). This companion tool as introduced in the next section builds upon the screening elements of STEADI, allowing for a more comprehensive falls risk assessment and intervention.

PHARMACIST ASSESSMENT FOR FALLS

Taking a stepwise approach, a pharmacist can conduct a comprehensive falls risk assessment. Six key steps are proposed.

Step 1

There are some key initial indicators, which quickly orient a pharmacist or other provider to increased falls risk (**Fig. 1**). Age is an independent risk factor for falling.[17] Falls risk increases with advancing age. Falls increase at times immediately preceding, during, or following a care transition.[7,8] Transitions are prime times for confusion, greater debilitation, communication gaps, and medication errors, which can contribute to falls. Knowledge about a patient's living arrangements provides valuable insight regarding the patient's support network and availability or lack of important at-home safety resources. It is important for pharmacists to ask older adults about alcohol and other substances of abuse. Substance use disorders are a frequently un-addressed cause of falls among the older adult population.[18] Pharmacists can use the power of observation to identify mobility-related falls risk factors, such as the presence of an assistive ambulation device (eg, cane, walker, or arm of a caregiver), unsteady gait, or difficulty standing or rising from a chair. In addition, there are other common general signs associated with falling for which the pharmacist and other practitioners should assess (**Box 2, Table 1**).

Step 2

The number one predictor of a fall is a previous fall.[19] It is rare unless there is injury for patients to voluntarily share the occurrence of a fall. Often what health professionals

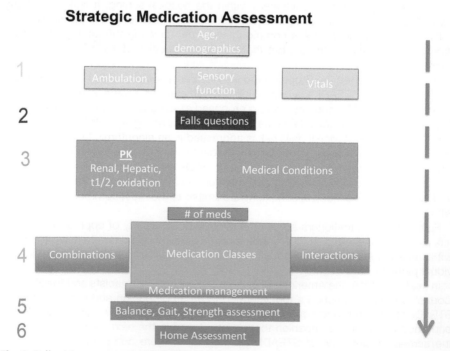

Fig. 1. Falls risk assessment algorithm

Box 2
Additional falls-related general signs or conditions

- Vital signs
  - Blood pressure: assess for hypotension or orthostatic hypotension
  - Heart rate: assess for any abnormal rate and rhythm
  - Temperature: assess for fever (infection >>> confusion >>> fall)
  - Pain: uncontrolled pain as distractor >>> falls

- Sensory function
  - Vision: use of assistive devices, last vision evaluation, impairments that cannot be corrected
  - Hearing: use of assistive devices, last hearing evaluation if any evidence of impairment
  - Taste/smell: impact on nutrition, strength, frailty
  - Touch: neuropathy, especially of the lower extremities

- Medication self-management—assess adherence, access, administration skills, and organization tool needs (mismanagement of medications >>> worsening of a falls-inducing medical condition and/or the occurrence of a falls-inducing adverse reaction)

---

would clearly define as a fall, patients will write-off as something other than a fall. "Oh, I didn't fall; I caught myself on the chair." For these reasons and others, it is important for pharmacists and other practitioners to ask about falls. Three key questions can be used to quickly screen for current falls risk and need for further assessment[14] (**Box 3**).

If a patient has experienced a fall, it is important to garner the patient's perspective as to the cause of the fall. At times, patients will be very uncertain as to the reason for their fall and claim "I don't know. All I know is the next minute I was on the floor." Other times patients may be able to speak to a specific cause: "my knee just gave out" or "I tripped over the living room rug" or "my chair tipped over when I was getting up." The more uncertainty as to the reason for the fall, the more likely there are to be causative factors completely unknown to the patient. This uncertainty will generally open up greater opportunities for assessment and patient education. However, just because the patient can point to a specific cause for their fall does not mean that the patient will not benefit from closer assessment and intervention. Falls are often multifactorial. A patient who seemingly fell due to tripping over clutter may have had their fall compounded by the presence of a balance-altering condition, FRID, or both.

Fear of falling alters how people live. Daily activities are limited or avoided; risk of isolation increases, and deconditioning can worsen.[20]

Step 3

There are several medical conditions that increase falls through physical function, neurologic, vascular, or pharmacokinetic changes. It is important for the pharmacist to educate patients regarding any falls-associated medical conditions as well as safety measures a patient can take to mitigate their risk (**Table 2**).

Step 4

Polypharmacy has been defined as 5 or more prescription medications.[74] Medication use in an aging population is a fine balance between evidence-based prescribing to sustain and enhance health and avoidance of inappropriate prescribing. Several tools have been designed and published to help guide appropriate prescribing. Some emphasize avoidance of medications with greater risk than efficacy.[75–78] Others emphasize inclusion of medications demonstrated to enhance health.[76] With advancing age often comes an accumulation of medical conditions and health issues.

Table 1
General assessment

General Patient Factors		
Age		
☐ Age over 65	☐ Age over 80	☐ Frail
Transition status		
☐ Pending transition	☐ Recent transition	
Living arrangements		
☐ Lives alone	☐ In-home care, full time	☐ In-home care, part time
☐ Lives with spouse or other	☐ Assisted living facility	☐ Skilled care facility
Substance use		
☐ Alcohol, _____ drinks per day	☐ Marijuana	☐ Other illicit substances
Vital signs		
Postural hypotension:	Pulse:	Pain:
☐ Systolic blood pressure (BP) falls ≥ −20 mm Hg	☐ Irregular	☐ Complaint of pain
	☐ <50 bpm	Pain location(s):
☐ Diastolic BP falls ≥ −10 mm Hg	Temperature:	Pain score _____ (0–10)
☐ Dizzy or lightheaded with standing	☐ Over 98.6°F	
Ambulation status		
☐ Cane	☐ Crutches	☐ Standard walker
☐ Front wheel walked	☐ Rollator	☐ Wheelchair
Sensory function		
Vision:	Hearing:	Feet/lower extremities:
☐ Acuity <20/40	☐ Hearing deficit	☐ Altered lower-extremity sensation
☐ Blurred vision	☐ Regular use hearing aid	☐ Foot pain
☐ No eye examination in last year	☐ Sporadic use hearing aid	☐ Bunion
☐ Corrected vision	Taste/smell:	☐ Hammer toe
☐ Regular use of glasses/contact lens	☐ Changes in taste	☐ Plantar fasciitis
☐ Sporadic use glasses/contacts	☐ Changes in smell	☐ Heel spur
		☐ Ingrown toenail
Medication self-management		
☐ Medications disorganized	☐ Evidence of adherence issues	

Box 3
Three quick screening questions for falls

1. Have you fallen in the past year?
   a. If yes, ask how many times and if there were any injuries.

2. Do you feel unsteady when standing or walking?

3. Do you worry about falling?

If the response is "yes" to any of these, then comprehensive assessment is warranted.

Data from Stevens JA, Phelan EA. Development of STEADI: a fall prevention resource for health care providers. Health Promot Pract 2013;14:710.

Polypharmacy might be a reflection of overall health, or it may be a trigger to identify higher risk of inappropriate prescribing.[79]

In some instances, especially when FRIDs are involved, falls risk can increase even with fewer than 5 prescribed medications.[80,81] This risk further increases in patients with more advanced age, use of ambulation assistive devices, and overall poorer health.[82,83]

Changing medication regimens is a source of confusion, error, and adverse effects. A recent medication change can be a flag for pharmacist intervention.

The medication assessment starts with number of medications, determination of any recent medication changes, and an awareness of medication-related problems that can increase falls risk (**Table 3**).

The next step of the medication assessment is to look for medication classes that increase falls risk. Most of these have central nervous system (CNS) depressant, anticholinergic, hypoglycemic, or hypotensive effects (**Table 4**).

Step 5

For further falls risk assessment, there are 3 quick and relatively simple gait, strength, and balance assessments that provide objective evidence of falls risk (**Box 4**).

Step 6

The final step is to know what falls risk factors are present in the home. For those residing in assisted living or skilled nursing facilities, there is a team of providers assessing these risks. For those not living in an institutional setting, an environmental assessment allows identification and reduction of additional risks (**Box 5**).

OPERATIONALIZING PHARMACIST-CONDUCTED FALLS ASSESSMENT

The vision for the profession of pharmacy by 2020 calls for an advanced role for pharmacists in all patient care settings. Pharmacists, as members of the patient's health care team, will take on greater roles "in promoting wellness, preventing disease and contributing to disease management."[131] Falls risk assessment by pharmacists is one such advanced role. However, the infrastructure and payment models for advanced pharmacist-provided services have been challenging at best if not seemingly insurmountable barriers at times.

The assessment described above takes time. How does a pharmacist work this type of comprehensive service into their existing daily duties? Which patients does one target for screening or for a more comprehensive assessment? Depending on the

Table 2
Medical conditions associated with falls risk

Medical Conditions	Caveats
Arrhythmia (eg, atrial fibrillation, a fib)	Any rhythm abnormality increases falls risk; a fib has higher mortality[21–23]
Arthritis (osteo, rheumatoid)	Osteoarthritis of lower extremities highest risk; over time, strength & flexibility decline[24–26]; rheumatic conditions associated with fatigue and added falls risk during flare[27,28]
Cardiovascular disease	Rate or rhythm disturbance, impaired oxygenation and stamina all increase risk[29]; syncope; myocardial infarction with atypical heralding symptoms[30,31]
Cerebellar ataxia	Gait variability and falls risk[32]
Cerebrovascular accident (CVA)/Stroke	CVA and associated sequelae can impact balance, physical function, ambulation[33–35]
Dementia	Impact of Alzheimer disease and other dementias multifactorial, including brain atrophy, declining frontal cognitive functions, impact on sleep cycles, falls associated with multitasking difficulty[36,37]
Depression	Common comorbidity with chronic conditions; negatively impacts motivation, concentration, and planning[38–41]
Hemophilia	Brain or muscle bleeds, bleed in the joint can impair mobility[42]; fear of injury can lead to decreased physical stamina and fitness; hemophilia with incontinence has even higher falls risk[43]
Impaired hepatic function	Impact on dosing; monitor AST, ALT, CYP450 enzymes; alcohol has negative impact on hepatic function and falls risk[44]; nonalcoholic fatty liver disease,[45] cirrhosis, hepatic encephalopathy with elevated ammonia levels associated with falls[46,47]
Impaired renal function	Renal impairment impacts clearance of medications, therapeutic and adverse effects; hemodialysis associated with falls risk[48,49]
Incontinence	Rush to bathroom, nocturia (with other risks of ambulating at night quickly in the dark with rapid standing not fully awake), urgency, urinary tract infections (UTIs) increase falls risk[50–52]
Infection (eg, UTI)	Confusion common symptom of infection; infections with most evidence of falls risk are UTI, bronchitic, pneumonia[53,54]
Lower extremity issue	Arthroplasty (especially first 1–3 d postoperative), neuropathy, injury, pain, physical changes, wounds, weakness all associated with falls (others); assure ambulation assistive device used correctly[55–62]
Malnutrition	Risk factors of muscle mass loss, weakness, associated cognitive decline, reduced concentration, sedation, reduced energy and stamina[63,64]
Multiple sclerosis	Annual fall rate near 60%; multifactorial[65,66]
Obesity	Associated with sedentary lifestyle, decreased strength, flexibility, stamina, muscle atrophy; may be associated with lower socioeconomic status, chronic health conditions, pain, anxiety, depression[67,68]
Parkinson disease	Orthostatic hypotension, gradually increasing imbalance, freezing, on/off phenomenon, impaired cognition[69,70]
Seizures	Syncopal and ictal episodes, especially if associated with loss of consciousness[71,72]; ictal bradyarrhythmias as a form of arrhythmogenic epilepsy[73]

Table 3
General medication assessment

Medication Review		
Number of medications (Rx, as needed, OTC, vitamin, supplement, herbal)	☐ ≥5	☐ ≥10
Recent medication regimen change	☐ Within last week	☐ Within last month
Falls risk medication-related problems detected:		
☐ Suboptimal dose[a] ☐ Interactions between medications, food, medical conditions ☐ Allergies and intolerances within current regimen	☐ Dose too high[b] ☐ Lacking medication therapy for all medication-requiring indications ☐ Unnecessary medication	☐ Safer evidence-based therapy available ☐ Difficulty administering medication[c]

[a] Suboptimal dose - check doses based on renal and hepatic function.
[b] Dose too high - causing adverse effects and/or unnecessary risk.
[c] Eye drops, inhalers, large dosage forms.

setting in which the pharmacist works, it may be wise to partner with others in carrying out various components of the assessment.

In the hospital, depending on patient data and falls metrics for the facility, it may be prudent to include a pharmacist in the assessment of any patient who is seen in the emergency department beause of a fall-related injury. The number one predictor of falling is a recent history of a fall.[19] Therefore, in the emergency department, if the causative factors are not initially and adequately addressed, another fall and subsequent emergency room visit or hospitalization is likely to occur. Inpatient pharmacists at the time of dispensing can flag FRIDs before initial administration, such that appropriate precautions can be put in place on the floor to prevent an in-hospital fall. When appropriate, safer alternatives can be recommended by the inpatient pharmacist. Before discharge, pharmacists can help provide patient education on appropriate use of medications and safety precautions to help minimize falls risk after hospitalization. In addition, pharmacists are important individuals to include on patient education committees, which may be responsible for designing or selecting falls risk education materials for patients and caregivers.

The long-term-care operational pharmacist can screen initial orders, on a skilled or assisted-living new patient admission, for FRIDs and alert the nursing and medical staff to not only the risk, but also potentially safer options. The consultant pharmacist in these postacute and long-term-care settings can review patient-specific falls-related information from the Minimum Data Set (MDS) 3.0,[132] as well as patient care notes, and participate in care planning to design a team-based approach to falls risk reduction.

In the outpatient setting, pharmacists who are embedded in ambulatory care practices have frequently been found to improve patient outcomes for diabetes, hypertension, hyperlipidemia, and anticoagulation services. More recently, pharmacists in collaboration with medical practices have become more involved in screening and preventative services, such as the MAWV.[133] A brief falls screening is part of the MAWV. Pharmacists can be instrumental in helping a medical practice conduct more comprehensive follow-up to problems detected during the wellness check. Pharmacists are especially beneficial for problems such as falls that are commonly known to be associated with medications.

Table 4
Medication review

Medication Class	Type	Effects
Anticholinergic	Anticholinergic (eg, oxybutynin, trihexiphenidyl, amitryptyline, antihistamines)	Dry eyes impact vision, dry mouth increases beverage consumption leading to frequent urination, CNS depression, constipation[84-86]
CNS depressant	Benzodiazepines (short or long t$_{1/2}$)	Consistent evidence of increased falls risk with all benzodiazepines; slow carefully monitored taper required for withdrawal of therapy[87-90]
	Antidepressants	Tricyclic agents have anticholinergic effects; selective serotonin reuptake inhibitors associated with fragility fractures and with falls; citalopram increases QTc interval; most require slow taper to withdraw[91-94]
	Sedative/hypnotics	Sleep cycles change with aging; typical requirement 7-8 h; agents impair gait, balance, equilibrium, can have amnestic effect, impaired motor vehicle operation[88,95]. consider melatonin 1-2 mg 1 h before bedtime[96]
	Antipsychotics/neuroleptics—typical or atypical	Typical agents primary mechanism with dopamine-associated with motor & extrapyramidal symptoms; atypical agents also associated with falls with mechanism more involving serotonin; risk similar among available atypical agents[97-99]
	Anticonvulsant	Associated with decreased bone density[100,101], use associated with falls and fractures[102]; risk of seizure increases with medication or dosing changes[103,104]
	Muscle relaxant	Not well-tolerated and limited evidence of efficacy; highly associated with falls[105,106]
	Opioids	CNS depressant effects,[107-111] constipation, taper slowly to withdraw with use over a few days[112]
	OTC: diphenhydramine, doxylamine	Sedating antihistamines and OTC sedatives are highly anticholinergic with CNS depressant effects[113]; use nonsedating antihistamines for allergies
Cardiovascular/endocrine	Antihypertensive/cardiovascular (CV) medications	Orthostatic hypotension, postural dizziness—assess orthostatic BP[114,115], include diet, weight management,[116] sleep apnea treatment in overall plan; goal is to treat to current guidelines to minimize CV risk while avoiding hypotension[117,118]
	Hypoglycemia agents	Insulin and sulfonylureas most associated with hypoglycemia; long-term metformin associated with B12 deficiency neuropathy[119-123]

Data from https://www.cms.gov/Medicare/Prescription-Drug-Coverage/PrescriptionDrugCovGenIn/Downloads/2016-Star-Ratings-User-Call-Slides-v2015_08_05.pdf. Accessed February 8, 2017.

Box 4
Gait, balance, strength

Timed Up and Go test ≥12 seconds[124–126]

30-second chair stand test below average score (scoring table with tool in STEADI)[127,128]

4-Stage balance test full tandem stance less than 10 seconds[129,130]

Observed gait problems or difficulty standing

Community pharmacists could establish an FRIDs component to their existing medication therapy management services or develop a separate service that could help build business for the pharmacy while improving the care of their patients. Because falling and falls injuries are frequently a cause of loss of independence, a

---

Box 5
Environmental assessment

Bathroom:

- Shower: lip or ledge to climb in
  - Surface, nonslip
  - Grab bars

- Toilet: raise seat if needed
  - Grab bars

- Space: wheelchair or walker accessible if needed

Bedroom:

- Bed: height, bed rail if needed

- Eyeglasses within reach

- Night light

- Accessibility to bathroom or bedside commode

Kitchen

- Ability to reach cabinets, pantry

- Safety of step stool if needed

Steps/stairs

- Height

- Sturdy rails

- Surface: nonslip or trip

- Adequate lighting

All rooms

- Open flow to ambulate between rooms and key spaces
  - Clutter and furniture out of path

- Electrical cords out of walking path

- Blind cords out of walking path

- Surfaces nonslip or trip

- Rugs removed or secured to floor

---

community-based falls-assessment service has the potential to help patients age in place more safely. Community pharmacists may want to set patient appointments for this type of service. Before an appointment, a technician could print out available and pertinent patient information for the pharmacist to review before or during the appointment. Community pharmacists could partner with aging services in the community as well as local care managers who could conduct initial falls screenings and refer appropriate patients to the pharmacist for a more comprehensive assessment. A community pharmacy may choose to train technicians or clerks to ask falls screening questions when interacting with patients at the time of medication pickup or delivery. Positive screenings could be reported back to the pharmacist for further action. Pharmacies could use electronic tablets preloaded with a falls screening question application. Patients or caregivers could self-screen and self-report to ask for further assessment.

SUMMARY

Falls frequently occur among the aging population, resulting in significant and sometimes fatal health consequences. Because of the aging of society, both the incidence and the cost of falls are anticipated to increase. Multiple factors, including medications, are commonly associated with falls in this patient population. Wherever older adults receive care, pharmacists are members of the patient health care team uniquely positioned to help assess and address falls risk. Comprehensive assessment such as the step-wise approach described within this article is needed to adequately identify and address multiple factors associated with falls in this population.

REFERENCES

1. Tromp AM, Pluijm SM, Smit JH, et al. Fall-risk screening test: a prospective study on predictors for falls in community-dwelling elderly. J Clin Epidemiol 2001; 54(8):837–44.
2. Centers for Disease Control and Prevention. Important facts about falls. Available at: http://www.cdc.gov/homeandrecreationalsafety/falls/adultfalls.html. Accessed June 19, 2016.
3. Tinetti ME, Williams CS. Falls, injuries due to falls, and the risk of admission to a nursing home. N Engl J Med 1997;337(18):1279–84.
4. Morbidity and Mortality Weekly Report. CDC National Health Report: leading causes of morbidity and mortality and associated behavioral risk and protective factors—United States, 2005–2013. Available at: http://www.cdc.gov/mmwr/preview/mmwrhtml/su6304a2.htm. Accessed June 20, 2016.
5. Centers for Disease Control and Prevention. Cost of falls among older adults. Available at: http://www.cdc.gov/homeandrecreationalsafety/falls/fallcost.html. Accessed June 19, 2016.
6. Stevens JA, Corso PS, Finkelstein EA, et al. The costs of fatal and nonfatal falls among older adults. Inj Prev 2006;12:290–5.
7. Stitt DM, Elliott DP, Thompson SN. Medication discrepancies identified at time of hospital discharge in a geriatric population. Am J Geriatr Pharmacother 2011; 9(4):234–40.
8. Mixon AS, Myers AP, Leak CL, et al. Characteristics associated with postdischarge medication errors. Mayo Clin Proc 2014;89(8):1042–51.
9. Casteel C, Blalock SJ, Ferreri S, et al. Implementation of a community pharmacy-based falls prevention program. Am J Geriatr Pharmacother 2011; 9(5):310–9.e2.

10. Mott DA, Martin B, Breslow R, et al. Impact of a medication therapy management intervention targeting medications associated with falling: results of a pilot study. J Am Pharm Assoc (2003) 2016;56(1):22–8.

11. Stevens JA, Ballesteros MF, Mack KA, et al. Gender differences in seeking care for falls in the aged medicare population. Am J Prev Med 2012;43:59–62.

12. RAND Corporation, Boston University School of Public Health, ECRI Institute. Agency for Healthcare Research and Quality. Preventing falls in hospitals: a toolkit for improving quality of care. Available at: http://www.ahrq.gov/professionals/systems/hospital/fallpxtoolkit/index.html. Accessed June 20, 2016.

13. Johns Hopkins falls risk assessment tool. Available at: http://www.hopkinsmedicine.org/institute_nursing/models_tools/Appendix%20A_JHFRAT.pdf. Accessed June 20, 2016.

14. Stevens JA, Phelan EA. Development of STEADI: a fall prevention resource for health care providers. Health Promot Pract 2013;14:706–14.

15. National Falls Prevention Resource Center. Center for Healthy Aging. National Council on Aging. STEADI implementation and partnering with health care. Available at: https://www.ncoa.org/wp-content/uploads/STEADI-Webinar-Slidedeck.pdf. Accessed June 20, 2016.

16. National Council on Aging. The 2015 Falls Free National Action Plan. Available at: https://www.ncoa.org/resources/2015-falls-free-national-falls-prevention-action-plan/. Accessed June 20, 2016.

17. Gillespie LD, Robertson MC, Gillespie WJ, et al. Interventions for preventing falls in older people living in the community. Cochrane Database Syst Rev 2012;(9):CD007146.

18. National Council on Alcoholism and Drug Dependence, Inc. An Invisible Epidemic: alcoholism and drug dependence among older adults. Available at: http://www.ncadd.org/images/stories/PDF/factsheet-alcoholismanddrugdependenceamongolderadults.pdf. Accessed June 20, 2016.

19. American Geriatrics Society. Prevention of falls in older persons: AGS/BGS clinical practice guidelines 2010. Available at: http://www.medcats.com/FALLS/frameset.htm. Accessed June 20, 2016.

20. Lachman ME, Howland J, Tennstedt S, et al. Fear of falling and activity restriction: the survey of activities and fear of falling in the elderly (SAFE). J Gerontol B Psychol Sci Soc Sci 1998;53:P43Y50.

21. O'Neal WT, Qureshi WT, Judd SE, et al. Effect of falls on frequency of atrial fibrillation and mortality risk (from the REasons for Geographic And Racial Differences in Stroke Study). Am J Cardiol 2015;116(8):1213–8.

22. Jansen S, Kenny RA, de Rooij SE, et al. Self-reported cardiovascular conditions are associated with falls and syncope in community-dwelling older adults. Age Ageing 2015;44(3):525–9.

23. Jansen S, Frewen J, Finucane C, et al. AF is associated with self-reported syncope and falls in a general population cohort. Age Ageing 2015;44(4):598–603.

24. Ng CT, Tan MP. Osteoarthritis and falls in the older person. Age Ageing 2013; 42(5):561–6.

25. Doré AL, Golightly YM, Mercer VS, et al. Lower-extremity osteoarthritis and the risk of falls in a community-based longitudinal study of adults with and without osteoarthritis. Arthritis Care Res (Hoboken) 2015;67(5):633–9.

26. Scott D, Blizzard L, Fell J, et al. Prospective study of self-reported pain, radiographic osteoarthritis, sarcopenia progression, and falls risk in community-dwelling older adults. Arthritis Care Res (Hoboken) 2012;64(1):30–7.

27. Brenton-Rule A, Dalbeth N, Bassett S, et al. The incidence and risk factors for falls in adults with rheumatoid arthritis: a systematic review. Semin Arthritis Rheum 2015;44(4):389–98.

28. Stanmore EK, Oldham J, Skelton DA, et al. Risk factors for falls in adults with rheumatoid arthritis: a prospective study. Arthritis Care Res (Hoboken) 2013; 65(8):1251–8.

29. Gnjidic D, Bennett A, Le Couteur DG, et al. Ischemic heart disease, prescription of optimal medical therapy and geriatric syndromes in community-dwelling older men: a population-based study. Int J Cardiol 2015;192:49–55.

30. Grosmaitre P, Le Vavasseur O, Yachouh E, et al. Significance of atypical symptoms for the diagnosis and management of myocardial infarction in elderly patients admitted to emergency departments. Arch Cardiovasc Dis 2013;106(11): 586–92.

31. Frisoli A Jr, Ingham SJ, Paes ÂT, et al. Frailty predictors and outcomes among older patients with cardiovascular disease: data from Fragicor. Arch Gerontol Geriatr 2015;61(1):1–7.

32. Schniepp R, Wuehr M, Schlick C, et al. Increased gait variability is associated with the history of falls in patients with cerebellar ataxia. J Neurol 2014;261(1): 213–23.

33. Jalayondeja C, Sullivan PE, Pichaiyongwongdee S. Six-month prospective study of fall risk factors identification in patients post-stroke. Geriatr Gerontol Int 2014; 14(4):778–85.

34. Tsang CS, Liao LR, Chung RC, et al. Psychometric properties of the Mini-Balance Evaluation Systems Test (MinI-BESTest) in community-dwelling individuals with chronic stroke. Phys Ther 2013;93(8):1102–15.

35. Minet LR, Peterson E, von Koch L, et al. Occurrence and predictors of falls in people with stroke: six-year prospective study. Stroke 2015;46(9):2688–90.

36. Mignardot JB, Beauchet O, Annweiler C, et al. Postural sway, falls, and cognitive status: a cross-sectional study among older adults. J Alzheimers Dis 2014; 41(2):431–9.

37. Epstein NU, Guo R, Farlow MR, et al. Medication for Alzheimer's disease and associated fall hazard: a retrospective cohort study from the Alzheimer's disease neuroimaging initiative. Drugs Aging 2014;31(2):125–9.

38. Stuart AL, Pasco JA, Jacka FN, et al. Falls and depression in men: a population-based study. Am J Mens Health 2015. [Epub ahead of print].

39. Kvelde T, Lord SR, Close JC, et al. Depressive symptoms increase fall risk in older people, independent of antidepressant use, and reduced executive and physical functioning. Arch Gerontol Geriatr 2015;60(1):190–5.

40. Launay C, De Decker L, Annweiler C, et al. Association of depressive symptoms with recurrent falls: a cross-sectional elderly population based study and a systematic review. J Nutr Health Aging 2013;17(2):152–7.

41. Lohman MC, Mezuk B, Dumenci L. Depression and frailty: concurrent risks for adverse health outcomes. Aging Ment Health 2015;1–10.

42. Fearn M, Hill K, Williams S, et al. Balance dysfunction in adults with haemophilia. Haemophilia 2010;16(4):606–14.

43. Sammels M, Vandesande J, Vlaeyen E, et al. Falling and fall risk factors in adults with haemophilia: an exploratory study. Haemophilia 2014;20(6):836–45.

44. Wadd S, Papadopoulos C. Drinking behaviour and alcohol-related harm amongst older adults: analysis of existing UK datasets. BMC Res Notes 2014; 7;741.

45. Bertolotti M, Lonardo A, Mussi C, et al. Nonalcoholic fatty liver disease and aging: epidemiology to management. World J Gastroenterol 2014;20(39): 14185–204.

46. Román E, Córdoba J, Torrens M, et al. Falls and cognitive dysfunction impair health-related quality of life in patients with cirrhosis. Eur J Gastroenterol Hepatol 2013;25(1):77–84.

47. Soriano G, Román E, Córdoba J, et al. Cognitive dysfunction in cirrhosis is associated with falls: a prospective study. Hepatology 2012;55(6):1922–30.

48. McAdams-DeMarco MA, Suresh S, Law A, et al. Frailty and falls among adult patients undergoing chronic hemodialysis: a prospective cohort study. BMC Nephrol 2013;14:224.

49. López-Soto PJ, De Giorgi A, Senno E, et al. Renal disease and accidental falls: a review of published evidence. BMC Nephrol 2015;16(1):176.

50. Luo X, Chuang CC, Yang E, et al. Prevalence, management and outcomes of medically complex vulnerable elderly patients with urinary incontinence in the United States. Int J Clin Pract 2015;69(12):1517–24.

51. Bresee C, Dubina ED, Khan AA, et al. Prevalence and correlates of urinary incontinence among older community-dwelling women. Female Pelvic Med Reconstr Surg 2014;20(6):328–33.

52. Godmaire GC, Grenier S, Tannenbaum C. An independent association between urinary incontinence and falls in chronic benzodiazepine users. J Am Geriatr Soc 2015;63(5):1035–7.

53. Infectious Diseases Society of America. Tripped up by a bug: infection may cause falls, especially in older people, study suggests. ScienceDaily 2015. Available at: www.sciencedaily.com/releases/2015/10/151009155255.htm. Accessed June 20, 2016.

54. Limpawattana P, Phungoen P, Mitsungnern T, et al. Atypical presentations of older adults at the emergency department and associated factors. Arch Gerontol Geriatr 2016;62:97–102.

55. Zak M, Krupnik S, Puzio G, et al. Assessment of functional capability and ongoing falls-risk in older institutionalized people after total hip arthroplasty for femoral neck fractures. Arch Gerontol Geriatr 2015;61(1):14–20.

56. Mallinson T, Leland NE, Chan TH. The need for uniform quality reporting across post-acute care rehabilitation settings: an examination of accidental falls. J Am Geriatr Soc 2015;63(1):195–7.

57. Matsumoto H, Okuno M, Nakamura T, et al. Incidence and risk factors for falling in patients after total knee arthroplasty compared to healthy elderly individuals. Yonago Acta Med 2014;57(4):137–45.

58. Swinkels A, Newman JH, Allain TJ. A prospective observational study of falling before and after knee replacement surgery. Age Ageing 2009;38(2):175–81.

59. Gell NM, Wallace RB, LaCroix AZ, et al. Mobility device use in older adults and incidence of falls and worry about falling: findings from the 2011-2012 national health and aging trends study. J Am Geriatr Soc 2015;63(5):853–9.

60. Toosizadeh N, Mohler J, Armstrong DG, et al. The influence of diabetic peripheral neuropathy on local postural muscle and central sensory feedback balance control. PLoS One 2015;10(8):e0135255.

61. Callaghan B, Kerber K, Langa KM, et al. Longitudinal patient-oriented outcomes in neuropathy: importance of early detection and falls. Neurology 2015;85(1): 71–9.

62. Johnson RL, Duncan CM, Ahn KS, et al. Fall-prevention strategies and patient characteristics that impact fall rates after total knee arthroplasty. Anesth Analg 2014;119(5):1113–8.

63. Westergren A, Hagell P, Sjödahl Hammarlund C. Malnutrition and risk of falling among elderly without home-help service–a cross sectional study. J Nutr Health Aging 2014;18(10):905–11.

64. Meijers JM, Halfens RJ, Neyens JC, et al. Predicting falls in elderly receiving home care: the role of malnutrition and impaired mobility. J Nutr Health Aging 2012;16(7):654–8.

65. Hoang PD, Cameron MH, Gandevia SC, et al. Neuropsychological, balance, and mobility risk factors for falls in people with multiple sclerosis: a prospective cohort study. Arch Phys Med Rehabil 2014;95(3):480–6.

66. Coote S, Finlayson M, Sosnoff JJ. Level of mobility limitations and falls status in persons with multiple sclerosis. Arch Phys Med Rehabil 2014;95(5):862–6.

67. Mitchell RJ, Lord SR, Harvey LA, et al. Obesity and falls in older people: mediating effects of disease, sedentary behavior, mood, pain and medication use. Arch Gerontol Geriatr 2015;60(1):52–8.

68. Mitchell RJ, Lord SR, Harvey LA, et al. Associations between obesity and overweight and fall risk, health status and quality of life in older people. Aust N Z J Public Health 2014;38(1):13–8.

69. Paul SS, Allen NE, Sherrington C, et al. Risk factors for frequent falls in people with Parkinson's disease. J Parkinsons Dis 2014;4(4):699–703.

70. Paul SS, Canning CG, Sherrington C, et al. Three simple clinical tests to accurately predict falls in people with Parkinson's disease. Mov Disord 2013;28(5): 655–62.

71. Nguyen-Michel VH, Bornand A, Balathazar AM, et al. Fall related to epileptic seizures in the elderly. Epileptic Disord 2015;17(3):287–91.

72. Homann B, Plaschg A, Grundner M, et al. The impact of neurological disorders on the risk for falls in the community dwelling elderly: a case-controlled study. BMJ Open 2013;3(11):e003367.

73. Kepez A, Erdogan O. Arrhythmogenic epilepsy and pacing need: a matter of controversy. World J Clin Cases 2015;3(10):872–5.

74. Gnjidic D, Hilmer SN, Blyth FM, et al. Polypharmacy cutoff and outcomes: five or more medicines were used to identify community-dwelling older men at risk of different adverse outcomes. J Clin Epidemiol 2012;65(9):989–95.

75. By the American Geriatrics Society 2015 Beers Criteria Update Expert Panel. American Geriatrics Society 2015 Updated Beers Criteria for potentially inappropriate medication use in older adults. J Am Geriatr Soc 2015;63(11):2227–46.

76. Gallagher P, Ryan C, Byrne S, et al. STOPP (Screening Tool of Older Person's Prescriptions) and START (Screening Tool to Alert doctors to Right Treatment). Consensus validation. Int J Clin Pharmacol Ther 2008;46(2):72–83.

77. Hill-Taylor B, Sketris I, Hayden J, et al. Application of the STOPP/START criteria: a systematic review of the prevalence of potentially inappropriate prescribing in older adults, and evidence of clinical, humanistic and economic impact. J Clin Pharm Ther 2013;38(5):360–72.

78. Fitzgerald LS, Hanlon JT, Shelton PS, et al. Reliability of a modified medication appropriateness index in ambulatory older persons. Ann Pharmacother 1997; 31(5):543–8.

79. Fried TR, O'Leary J, Towle V, et al. Health outcomes associated with polypharmacy in community-dwelling older adults: a systematic review. J Am Geriatr Soc 2014;62(12):2261–72.

80. Laflamme L, Monárrez-Espino J, Johnell K, et al. Type, number or both? A population-based matched case-control study on the risk of fall injuries among older people and number of medications beyond fall-inducing drugs. PLoS One 2015;10(3):e0123390.

81. Helgadóttir B, Laflamme L, Monárrez-Espino J, et al. Medication and fall injury in the elderly population; do individual demographics, health status and lifestyle matter? BMC Geriatr 2014;14:92.

82. Ham AC, Swart KM, Enneman AW, et al. Medication-related fall incidents in an older, ambulant population: the B-PROOF study. Drugs Aging 2014;31(12): 917–27.

83. Thorell K, Ranstad K, Midlöv P, et al. Is use of fall risk-increasing drugs in an elderly population associated with an increased risk of hip fracture, after adjustment for multimorbidity level: a cohort study. BMC Geriatr 2014;14:131.

84. Richardson K, Bennett K, Maidment ID, et al. Use of medications with anticholinergic activity and self-reported injurious falls in older community-dwelling adults. J Am Geriatr Soc 2015;63(8):1561–9.

85. Landi F, Dell'Aquila G, Collamati A, et al. Anticholinergic drug use and negative outcomes among the frail elderly population living in a nursing home. J Am Med Dir Assoc 2014;15(11):825–9.

86. Crispo JA, Willis AW, Thibault DP, et al. Associations between anticholinergic burden and adverse health outcomes in Parkinson disease. PLoS One 2016; 11(3):e0150621.

87. de Vries OJ, Peeters G, Elders P, et al. The elimination half-life of benzodiazepines and fall risk: two prospective observational studies. Age Ageing 2013; 42(6):764–70.

88. Allain H, Bentué-Ferrer D, Polard E, et al. Postural instability and consequent falls and hip fractures associated with use of hypnotics in the elderly: a comparative review. Drugs Aging 2005;22(9):749–65.

89. Guaiana G, Barbui C. Discontinuing benzodiazepines: best practices. Epidemiol Psychiatr Sci 2016;25(3):214–6.

90. Darker CD, Sweeney BP, Barry JM, et al. Psychosocial interventions for benzodiazepine harmful use, abuse or dependence. Cochrane Database Syst Rev 2015;(5):CD009652.

91. Sultana J, Spina E, Trifirò G. Antidepressant use in the elderly: the role of pharmacodynamics and pharmacokinetics in drug safety. Expert Opin Drug Metab Toxicol 2015;11(6):883–92.

92. Boyce RD, Handler SM, Karp JF, et al. Age-related changes in antidepressant pharmacokinetics and potential drug-drug interactions: a comparison of evidence-based literature and package insert information. Am J Geriatr Pharmacother 2012;10(2):139–50.

93. Coupland CA, Dhiman P, Barton G, et al. A study of the safety and harms of antidepressant drugs for older people: a cohort study using a large primary care database. Health Technol Assess 2011;15(28):1–202, iii–iv.

94. Kerse N, Flicker L, Pfaff JJ, et al. Falls, depression and antidepressants in later life: a large primary care appraisal. PLoS One 2008;3(6):e2423.

95. Gunja N. In the Zzz zone: the effects of Z-drugs on human performance and driving. J Med Toxicol 2013;9(2):163–71.

96. Vural EM, van Munster BC, de Rooij SE. Optimal dosages for melatonin supplementation therapy in older adults: a systematic review of current literature. Drugs Aging 2014;31(6):441–51.

97. Chatterjee S, Chen H, Johnson ML, et al. Risk of falls and fractures in older adults using atypical antipsychotic agents: a propensity score-adjusted, retrospective cohort study. Am J Geriatr Pharmacother 2012;10(2):83–94.
98. Mehta S, Chen H, Johnson ML, et al. Risk of falls and fractures in older adults using antipsychotic agents: a propensity-matched retrospective cohort study. Drugs Aging 2010;27(10):815–29.
99. Lavsa SM, Fabian TJ, Saul MI, et al. Influence of medications and diagnoses on fall risk in psychiatric inpatients. Am J Health Syst Pharm 2010;67(15):1274–80.
100. Gold PW, Pavlatou MG, Michelson D, et al. Chronic administration of anticonvulsants but not antidepressants impairs bone strength: clinical implications. Transl Psychiatry 2015;5:e576.
101. Carbone LD, Johnson KC, Robbins J, et al. Antiepileptic drug use, falls, fractures, and BMD in postmenopausal women: findings from the women's health initiative (WHI). J Bone Miner Res 2010;25(4):873–81.
102. Shiek Ahmad B, Hill KD, O'Brien TJ, et al. Falls and fractures in patients chronically treated with antiepileptic drugs. Neurology 2012;79(2):145–51.
103. Saengsuwan J, Laohasiriwong W, Boonyaleepan S, et al, Integrated Epilepsy Research Group. Seizure-related vehicular crashes and falls with injuries for people with epilepsy (PWE) in northeastern Thailand. Epilepsy Behav 2014; 32:49–54.
104. Classen S, Crizzle AM, Winter SM, et al. Evidence-based review on epilepsy and driving. Epilepsy Behav 2012;23(2):103–12.
105. Spence MM, Shin PJ, Lee EA, et al. Risk of injury associated with skeletal muscle relaxant use in older adults. Ann Pharmacother 2013;47(7–8):993–8.
106. IBillups SJ, Delate T, Hoover B. Injury in an elderly population before and after initiating a skeletal muscle relaxant. Ann Pharmacother 2011;45(4):485–91.
107. Pergolizzi J, Böger RH, Budd K, et al. Opioids and the management of chronic severe pain in the elderly: consensus statement of an International Expert Panel with focus on the six clinically most often used World Health Organization Step III opioids (buprenorphine, fentanyl, hydromorphone, methadone, morphine, oxycodone). Pain Pract 2008;8(4):287–313.
108. Söderberg KC, Laflamme L, Möller J. Newly initiated opioid treatment and the risk of fall-related injuries. A nationwide, register-based, case-crossover study in Sweden. CNS Drugs 2013;27(2):155–61.
109. O'Neil CK, Hanlon JT, Marcum ZA. Adverse effects of analgesics commonly used by older adults with osteoarthritis: focus on non-opioid and opioid analgesics. Am J Geriatr Pharmacother 2012;10(6):331–42.
110. Rolita L, Spegman A, Tang X, et al. Greater number of narcotic analgesic prescriptions for osteoarthritis is associated with falls and fractures in elderly adults. J Am Geriatr Soc 2013;61(3):335–40.
111. Dowell D, Haegerich TM, Chou R. CDC guideline for prescribing opioids for chronic pain—United States, 2016. MMWR Recomm Rep 2016;65:1–49.
112. Hao J, Lucido D, Cruciani RA. Potential impact of abrupt opioid therapy discontinuation in the management of chronic pain: a pilot study on patient perspective. J Opioid Manag 2014;10(1):9–20.
113. Albert SM, Roth T, Toscani M, et al. Sleep health and appropriate use of OTC sleep aids in older adults—recommendations of a Gerontological Society of America Workgroup. Gerontologist 2015. [Epub ahead of print].
114. Zia A, Kamaruzzaman SB, Tan MP. Blood pressure lowering therapy in older people: does it really cause postural hypotension or falls? Postgrad Med 2015;127(2):186–93.

115. Mills P, Gray D, Krassioukov A. Five things to know about orthostatic hypotension and aging. J Am Geriatr Soc 2014;62(9):1822–3.
116. Butt DA, Harvey PJ. Benefits and risks of antihypertensive medications in the elderly. J Intern Med 2015;278(6):599–626.
117. Tinetti ME, Han L, Lee DS, et al. Antihypertensive medications and serious fall injuries in a nationally representative sample of older adults. JAMA Intern Med 2014;174(4):588–95.
118. Lipsitz LA, Habtemariam D, Gagnon M, et al. Reexamining the effect of antihypertensive medications on falls in old age. Hypertension 2015;66(1):183–9.
119. Lapane KL, Jesdale BM, Dubé CE, et al. Sulfonylureas and risk of falls and fractures among nursing home residents with type 2 diabetes mellitus. Diabetes Res Clin Pract 2015;109(2):411–9.
120. Lapane KL, Yang S, Brown MJ, et al. Sulfonylureas and risk of falls and fractures: a systematic review. Drugs Aging 2013;30(7):527–47.
121. Kachroo S, Kawabata H, Colilla S, et al. Association between hypoglycemia and fall-related events in type 2 diabetes mellitus: analysis of a U.S. commercial database. J Manag Care Spec Pharm 2015;21(3):243–53.
122. Signorovitch JE, Macaulay D, Diener M, et al. Hypoglycaemia and accident risk in people with type 2 diabetes mellitus treated with non-insulin antidiabetes drugs. Diabetes Obes Metab 2013;15(4):335–41.
123. Berlie HD, Garwood CL. Diabetes medications related to an increased risk of falls and fall-related morbidity in the elderly. Ann Pharmacother 2010;44(4):712–7.
124. Bohannon RW. Reference values for the timed up and go test: a descriptive meta-analysis. J Geriatr Phys Ther 2006;29(2):64–8.
125. Herman T, Giladi N, Hausdorff JM. Properties of the 'timed up and go' test: more than meets the eye. Gerontology 2011;57:203–10.
126. Viccaro LJ, Perera S, Studenski SA. Is timed up and go better than gait speed in predicting health, function and falls in older adults? J Am Geriatr Soc 2011;59:887–92.
127. MacFarlane DJ, Chou KL, Cheng YH, et al. Validity and normative data for thirty-second chair stand test in elderly community-dwelling Hong Kong Chinese. Am J Hum Biol 2006;18:418–21.
128. Rikli RE, Jones CJ. Functional fitness normative scores for community-residing older adults, ages 60-94. J Aging Phys Act 1999;7:162–81.
129. Scott V, Votova K, Scanlan A, et al. Multifactorial and functional mobility assessment tools for fall risk among older adults in community, home-support, long-term and acute care settings. Age Ageing 2007;36:130–9.
130. Guralnik JM, Simonsick EM, Ferrucci L, et al. A short physical performance battery assessing lower extremity function: association with self-reported disability and prediction of mortality and nursing home admission. J Gerontol 1994;49(2):M85–94.
131. International Pharmaceutical Federation. 2020 vision: FIP's vision, mission and strategic plan. Available at: https://www.fip.org/files/fip/strategic%20plan%20no%20annexes.pdf. Accessed June 20, 2016.
132. Centers for Medicare and Medicaid Services. Long-term care facility resident assessment instrument 3.0 user's manual, version 1.13. Available at: https://www.cms.gov/Medicare/Quality-Initiatives-Patient-Assessment-Instruments/NursingHomeQualityInits/Downloads/MDS-30-RAI-Manual-V113.pdf. Accessed June 20, 2016.
133. Warshany K, Sherrill CH, Cavanaugh J, et al. Medicare annual wellness visits conducted by a pharmacist in an internal medicine clinic. Am J Health Syst Pharm 2014;71(1):44–9.

Medication Reconciliation in Long-Term Care and Assisted Living Facilities

Opportunity for Pharmacists to Minimize Risks Associated with Transitions of Care

Linda G. Gooen, PharmD, MS[a,b,*]

KEYWORDS

- Medication reconciliation • Transitions of care • Long-term care
- Adverse drug events • Electronic health records • Medication regimen review
- Polypharmacy

KEY POINTS

- Transitions of care (TOC) process involves pharmacists and other members of the health care team who are in a position to collect, review, and analyze medications lists to help improve health care outcomes.
- Medical, pharmacy, and health care organizations continue to advocate the involvement of pharmacists in the TOC process.
- Medication reconciliation is a complex process especially when providing care to elderly population due to increased medication use, the movement of the patient from one health care setting to another, the number of acute and chronic illnesses, and the intervention of multiple health care providers in different facilities.
- Because of the need for more frequent medication regimen reviews for patient stays under 30 days, the use of electronic health records (EHRs) can provide many benefits; however, many long-term care (LTC) and assisted living (AL) facilities have not yet instituted computerized systems.
- Clear financial incentives are currently limited and not fully directed toward the medication reconciliation process, which can ultimately reduce overall health care costs and improve outcomes.

[a] Gooen Consulting, LLC, Basking Ridge, NJ 07920, USA; [b] Pharmacy Practice and Administration, Ernest P. Mario School of Pharmacy, Rutgers University, New Brunswick, NY 08854, USA
* Gooen Consulting, LLC, Basking Ridge, NJ 07920.
E-mail address: Linda_Gooen@alumni.rutgers.edu

Clin Geriatr Med 33 (2017) 225–239
http://dx.doi.org/10.1016/j.cger.2017.01.006

INTRODUCTION

Medication reconciliation is a patient safety issue that is considered an integral part of good medical care. The TOC process involves pharmacists and other members of the health care team who are in a position to collect, review, and analyze medication lists to help improve health care outcomes. Pharmacists work in various health care settings that allow access to medical records in which pharmacists not only can review medication lists but also the latest medical clinical information that correlates to rational medication use. From these reviews, pharmacists can take steps to minimize adverse drug events (ADEs) and increase medication safety.

Patients often have changes made to their medications at various points in their lives. These changes can occur on hospital admission, transfer to different units within the same or different hospitals, or transfer to an LTC or AL facility or to home. Health care providers, mainly prescribers, may be not be cognizant of the most recent medication changes. These changes, whether intentional or unintentional, may result in omissions, unnecessary duplicate therapies, or incorrect dosing of medications.

A complicating factor often involves formulary considerations, which often require changes in a patient's baseline therapy prior to admission in the LTC or AL facility. This creates the potential for confusion for the patient and the nursing staff of the facility. Clear communication about newer medication changes may not occur, which can lead to medication errors and adverse events.

The consideration and responsibilities for patient safety and medication reconciliation involve several disciplines from health care practitioners to the administrators and leaders of LTC, AL, and hospital facilities. Empowerment of patients, patients' families, and caregivers when moving from one setting to another should always be encouraged because transition from one setting to another may occur frequently as a patient's medical status changes, and every transition has the potential to cause medication-related problems.

STATISTICS

Adverse drug reactions (ADRs) are the sixth leading cause of death in the United States.[1] The risk for developing an ADR is estimated to be 20%. As people age, medication use generally increases. Elderly patients who experience an ADR have a risk of hospitalization of approximately 10.7% compared with a risk of 5.3% for the general population.[2]

More than 770,00 people are injured or die each year in hospitals from ADEs.[3,4] It is estimated that these events may cost up to $5.6 million each year per hospital.[5,6]

In a prospective study of patients who used at least 4 prescription medications, more than 53% of unintended medication discrepancies were reported at the time of hospital admission[7]; 38.6% of these unintended discrepancies had the potential to cause moderate to severe discomfort or clinical deterioration.

In another study by Mark Beers and colleagues,[8] known for the development of the Beers Criteria, 60% of patients had at least 1 medication discrepancy error from the hospital medication history in comparison to the written record obtained from the patient. Failure to record use in the hospital was reported, and these errors may adversely affect clinical care.[8]

Adults over the age of 65 years are twice as likely as younger adults to visit emergency departments for ADEs.[9] ADEs include allergic reactions, undesirable pharmacologic or idiosyncratic effects at recommended doses, unintentional overdoses, and secondary effects that include falls and choking.[10,11]

Four medication classes and medications are listed as causing the greatest risk of increased hospitalizations for the elderly: warfarin (33.3%); insulins (13.9%); oral anti-platelet agents, which include aspirin and clopidogrel (13.3%); and oral hypoglycemic agents (10.7%). Other common drugs recognized by the Centers for Disease Control and Prevention include phenytoin and digoxin.[12]

The increase in deaths due to drug overdose in the population ages 65 and older was 7.7% from 2013 to 2014.[13] Currently, particular attention is drawn to drug overdose deaths that include opioid use.

GUIDING PRINCIPLES OF MEDICATION RECONCILIATION

Medication reconciliation is the process of creating the most accurate list possible of all medications a patient is taking, according to the Institute for Healthcare Improvement.[14] This includes the drug name, dosage, frequency, and route so that all the correct medications are listed to prevent unintended changes or omissions of medications at all transition points.

The Agency for Healthcare Research and Quality, US Department of Health and Human Services, and the World Health Organization have developed guiding principles to medication reconciliation. They are listed in **Table 1**.[15,16] The elements of these principles are pertinent to medication reconciliation in LTC and AL facilities.

Table 1
Comparing guiding principles for designing a successful medication reconciliation process

Agency for Healthcare Research and Quality http://www.ahrq.gov/professionals/quality-patient-safety/patient-safety-resources/resources/match/match3.html	World Health Organization http://www.who.int/patientsafety/implementation/solutions/high5s/h5s-sop.pdf
Develop a single medication list ("One Source of Truth"), shared by all disciplines for documenting a patient's current medications.	An up-to-date and accurate patient medication list is essential to ensure safe prescribing in any setting.
Clearly define roles and responsibilities for each discipline involved in medication reconciliation.	A formal structured process for reconciling medications should be in place across all interfaces of care.
Standardize and simplify the medication reconciliation process throughout the organization, and eliminate unnecessary redundancies.	Medication reconciliation on admission is the foundation for reconciliation throughout the episode of care.
Make the right thing to do the easiest thing to do within the patterns of normal practice.	Medication reconciliation is integrated into existing processes for medication management and patient flow.
Develop effective prompts or reminders for consistent behavior if true forcing functions (ie, required reconciliation step presented to the physician during admission order entry within an EHR) are not possible.	The process of medication reconciliation is one of shared accountability with staff aware of their roles and responsibilities.
Educate patients and their families or caregivers on medication reconciliation and the important role they play in the process.	Patients and families are involved in medication reconciliation.
Ensure process design meets all pertinent local laws or regulatory requirements.	Staff responsible for reconciling medicines are trained to take a best possible medication history and reconcile medicines.

FOCUS ON TRANSITION OF CARE FROM HEALTH CARE ORGANIZATIONS

The focus on the issue of TOC has been intensified within the past few years for health care providers and to the public. This issue has been identified and advocated by national interdisciplinary organizations, including the National Transitions of Care Coalition[17] and The Joint Commission.[18] The Joint Commission introduced medication reconciliation as a National Patient Safety Goal in 2005 and this Safety Goal has been updated to include the risk points of medication reconciliation that include coordinating information during transitions in care both within and outside of the organization, resident education on safe medication use, and communication with other providers.[19]

The American College of Physicians, Society of Hospital Medicine, Society of General Internal Medicine, American Geriatrics Society, and more than 30 organizations that represent pharmacists, nurses, and patient groups convened to develop and issue a Transitions of Care Consensus Policy Statement. This statement addresses gaps in communication during transitions between inpatient and outpatient settings.[20]

Pharmacy, medical, and health care organizations continue to advocate the involvement of pharmacists in the TOC process. Several programs about TOC have been sponsored through the American Society of Consultant Pharmacists and the Academy of Managed Care Pharmacy. Special interest groups have been formed by the American Society of Health-System Pharmacists,[21] the American Pharmacists Association,[22] and the American Geriatrics Society.[23]

GOVERNMENT FOCUS OF TRANSITION OF CARE IN SKILLED NURSING FACILITIES

TOC involves an increased risk for complications and ADEs for the patient. In particular, the issue of medication reconciliation for LTC facilities has been heightened by the interest and publication of Centers for Medicare & Medicaid Services (CMS) proposed rules initially issued in the *Federal Register* on July 16, 2015. Two sections of the proposed rule addressed the issues of effective communication between care providers and discharge planning.[24]

According to the proposed rules, the transferring facility must provide the necessary information to a resident's receiving provider, whether it is an acute care hospital, an LTC hospital, a psychiatric facility, another LTC facility, a hospice, a home health agency, or another community-based provider or practitioner. Timely and accurate clinical information exchange must follow patients across settings of care and to the health care providers. In addition, the LTC megarule addresses discharge planning that includes the reconciliation of all predischarge medications with postdischarge prescription and over-the-counter medications.

The universal transfer form is currently mandated in New Jersey and in other states. This form is required to be used to include patient information during periods of movement from one facility to another.[25] This form includes clinical and patient care information with attached medication-related documents, including the medication administration record (MAR), the treatment administration record, and physician order sheets.

Case study 1 in **Box 1** demonstrates that several issues need to be addressed at readmission to a skilled nursing facility (SNF). These include addressing drug interactions, duration of therapies, a review of dosage formulations, and administration of medications at best administration times.

Warfarin is considered one of the medications that increases the risk of hospitalization due to serious side effects from inappropriate dosing and drug interactions. Reported drug interactions with warfarin may occur due to amoxicillin/clavulanate, atorvastatin, and celecoxib.

Box 1
Case study 1

PM, an 89-year-old man with mild dysphagia and with no known drug allergies, was admitted back to the facility from a 1-day hospitalization due to recent fall, increased confusion, and dysphagia. He was readmitted after medication reconciliation by nursing.

Medications

Amoxicillin/clavulanate, 875 mg/125 mg bid

Atorvastatin, 40 mg hs

Warfarin, 5 mg hs

Omeprazole, 20 mg bid

Lisinopril, 2.5 mg hs

Lanoxin, 0.125 mg daily

Metoprolol, 12.5 mg daily

Fiber tabs, 1350 mg bid

Saccharomyces boulardii, 250 mg bid

Neurontin, 600 mg tid

Celecoxib, 200 mg daily

Furosemide, 20 mg daily

Diclofenac gel 1%, tid

Tamsulosin, 0.4 mg hs

Acetaminophen, 1 g bid

Laboratory results

PT/INR: 18.9/2.37 (on readmission)
   Glucose: 90
   Serum urea nitrogen: 14
   Sodium: 138
   Potassium: 4.8
   Glomerular filtration rate estimate: 96.9
   Serum digoxin: 0.6
   Hemoglobin: 12.5
   Hematocrit: 37.3
   Creatinine: 0.8
   Culture and sensitivity urine: *E coli* >100,000 count; sensitive to amoxicillin/clavulanate potassium

---

On transfer to an SNF, the duration of the antibiotic therapy, amoxicillin/clavulanate, is omitted from the medication list and needs to be obtained. The warfarin order should also note the time period when the current dose needs to be reevaluated from prothrombin time (PT)/international normalized ratio (INR) laboratory updates.

Because the resident has dysphagia, the dosage formulation of each medication must be reviewed to determine if the tablets are crushable. The pharmacist must clarify the formulation of metoprolol—whether the long-acting tablet must be administered or the tartrate (crushable) formulation can be substituted.

Obtaining the medication list on readmission requires further scrutiny to determine if the resident had other medications prior to discharge from the hospital. In this case, the resident had a donepezil order that was not included. On verification, it was determined by the prescriber that the donepezil order had to be reinstated.

THE PROCESS OF MEDICATION RECONCILIATION FROM HOSPITAL TO NURSING HOME AND/OR ASSISTED LIVING

Initially, the process for medication reconciliation seems simple and straightforward: obtaining a patient's preadmission medication on admission and reconciling the patient's current medication list with the medications ordered, as illustrated in **Fig. 1**. When examining the process, however, several factors must be considered when a patient moves from a hospital to a nursing home.

When reviewing the flowchart, no standardized consistent process for medication reconciliation is evident. Communication between nursing, prescriber, and dispensing pharmacist and consultant pharmacist may be lacking. Frequently, changes to therapy can be buried in the progress notes or in the charts from the hospital, increasing the likelihood of medication errors. This may also cause inaccuracies in the medication history.

As a result, increased time is spent to clarify discrepancies due to inconsistent prescriber documentation as described in Agency for Healthcare Research and Quality Medications at Transitions and Clinical Handoffs (MATCH) Toolkit for Medication Reconciliation.[26]

MEDICATION HISTORY PROCESS QUESTIONS

Many breakdowns in the communication of accurate medication from one setting to another is a concern. At times the duplication of orders written as generics versus brand names is noted. Formulary considerations from hospital to LTC may cause the change of one medication to another.

The follow-up on discrepancies may also be lacking. Most of the burden of discovering medication discrepancies in the LTC/AL setting is done by nursing because nursing staff is on site, has the most contact with patients, and is available in the facility 24 hours per day. Clarification of orders takes time and documenting the resolution of the discrepancy may not occur.

COMMON BARRIERS TO MEDICATION RECONCILIATION

Several barriers cause difficulty and inefficiencies in accessing and sharing complete medication information through the health care settings.

Medication reconciliation takes time. The medication orders need to be verified by checking for omissions, for inappropriate continuation of medications, and for

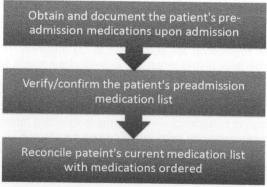

Fig. 1. Simplified medication process.

reviewing the physician progress notes against the medications that were ordered. Contacting the prescriber who is not on site at the facility and obtaining a response to verify the orders does not easily occur. Difficulty in communicating with the prescriber depends on the time of the day, the day of the week, and on holidays.

Clarification of medication orders may delay delivery of medications by the pharmacy. Cutoff times for pharmacy orders from the facility have to be met to ensure timely access of medications for administration to the patient.

The physician who treated the patient at home or in the hospital often is not the same physician in the nursing home or in the AL home. Because of changes of the prescribers and other health care providers and the medication history from the previous prescriber may not be complete, the risk of medication errors is most likely to increase.

ELECTRONIC HEALTH RECORDS

The use of EHRs can have a positive impact on patient safety if implemented and used by the facility. This depends on the software system, the use by health care disciplines, and the maintenance of the system. According to the American Health Information Management Association, EHRs can provide many beneficial benefits.[27]

Using an integrated pharmacy database can reduce medication errors. A computerized system can provide alerts to allergies, drug interactions, adverse effects, and billing information. EHRs can be programmed to insert appropriate drug administration times and other pertinent adjuvant information into the MAR.

Improved clinical documentation may improve clinical decision making. EHRs are able to include pertinent clinical information into specific sections that can be easily obtained by the prescriber and other health care team members. Physician orders can be easily correlated to the MARs, which minimizes the risk for errors.

Most importantly, EHRs can be programmed to allow electronic health information exchange. The TOC information between health care providers and facilities at admission, discharge, or transfer can be improved by the timely sharing of this information.

Unfortunately, nursing homes lag behind other providers, such as hospitals and physicians, in EHRs. In a study surveying New York State nursing homes between February 2013 and May 2013 and comparing the results to the same survey administered in 2012, researchers surveyed 472 nursing homes, of which 56.3% of homes had EHRs.[28] There was only a 7.7% increase in EHRs by nursing homes between February 2013 and May 2013. As of 2013 the electronic functionalities were minimum data set reporting, financial management, and patient demographics. Computerized provider order entry was available in 56.9% of facilities and clinical notes were available in 51.5% of those facilities that had EHRs.

The main barriers to nursing home EHRs were costs, lack of financial incentives, and lack of technical staff in LTC and AL facilities. Implementing EHRs requires a substantial initial investment and additional costs for future upgrades and maintenance.[29]

The proposed CMS rules issued on July 16, 2015, require LTC facilities to send patient care summaries to the nursing facility receiving the patient during transfer. The new rules do not require EHRs, but the process and the language of the regulations promote adoption and use of computerized systems.[24]

MEDICATION REGIMEN REVIEWS DURING TRANSITION OF CARE BY THE CONSULTANT PHARMACIST

Many LTC facilities expanded into the field of subacute care for those patients who need rehabilitation after hospitalization. Subacute care is defined as comprehensive inpatient care designed for someone who has an acute illness, injury, or exacerbation of a disease process, such as chronic obstructive pulmonary disease, pneumonia, or joint replacement.[30,31] Typically, subacute care serves to transition patients from the hospital to home. Rehabilitation services and specialized care for certain conditions, including stroke, diabetes, and postsurgical care, may be provided by the LTC facility.

According to the State Operations Manual, the facility is expected to have a proactive, systematic, and effective approach to monitoring, reporting, and acting on the effects, risks, and adverse consequences of medications of patients who stay under 30 days or who have a change in medical condition.[24] This is applicable to all residents, including those residents who have respite, end-of-life, or hospice care and those residents who have an anticipated stay of under 30 days.

Because the patients in subacute care facilities within the LTC facilities are shorter-stay patients, generally a few days to a maximum of 100 days, the consultant pharmacist needs to visit the facility more than once per month or to review the drug regimen review off-site. Off-site reviews can be managed through secure faxes or through secured computer systems.

Potential findings of discrepancies during off-site drug regimen review are found in **Box 2**. These findings are taken from the State Operations Manual, Appendix PP.[24]

The case study 2 in **Box 3** study emphasizes the need for the consultant pharmacist to review the past LTC discharge to the hospital form in addition to the transfer order from the hospital. According to the prescribing formation for rivastigmine (Exelon patch), for treatment interruption longer than 3 days, retitrate dosage starting at 4.6 mg/24 h.[32] This was communicated to the prescriber and the order was changed.

The patient is noted to be allergic to codeine. Hydrocodone is a semisynthetic opiate. The consultant pharmacist along with nursing have an obligation to report a possible cross-sensitivity reaction although most patients do not have true opioid allergies. Codeine is an opioid most commonly associated with pseudoallergy; therefore, careful monitoring for a reaction to hydrocodone may be justified.[33]

Pain management should be carefully reviewed. The patient is routinely taking 1300 mg of acetaminophen daily. The use of hydrocodone/acetaminophen prior to admission and on readmission needs to be reviewed to determine if pain is being managed. Further evaluation should be made to determine if the patient is requiring

---

Box 2
Potential findings of the drug regimen review during medication reconciliation

- Allergies and potential for cross-sensitivity reactions
- Omissions
- Duplication of therapy
- Drug-drug interactions
- Potential adverse effects
- Dose and dosing intervals
- Administration times
- Fall precaution
- Diagnosis corresponding to medication therapy
- Laboratory orders or monitoring parameters
- Miscommunication during the transition from one team of care providers to another

---

Box 3
Case study 2

RV, an 87-year-old man with a diagnosis of dementia with behavioral disturbances, sleep disturbances, sleep apnea, generalized pain, aortic valve disorders, and anxiety was readmitted to SNF after a week stay from the hospital. He is allergic to codeine.

Medications

Memantine hydrochloride, 10 mg bid

Rivastigmine transdermal patch, 9.5 mg/24 h to upper back in the morning, replace daily

Warfarin, 3 mg daily

Melatonin, 3 mg daily

Acetaminophen, 650 mg bid

Ativan gel, 0.25 mg bid to skin prn anxiety

Hydrocodone/acetaminophen, 5/325 1 tablet q4h prn pain

Milk of magnesia, 30 mL daily prn constipation

Vitamin B complex hs

Phosphatidylserine 100 capsule, 1 capsule in the morning

Ubiquinol 200 mg, daily at lunch

Resveratrol, 1 capsule daily at lunch

Pycnogenol, 1 capsule daily

Curcumin, 1 capsule daily at lunch

Vitamin D$_2$, 50,000 U monthly

Note: the rivastigmine patch was not on the hospital transfer order sheet; however, after contacting the prescriber, the patch was to continue.

---

more than 3000 mg of acetaminophen per day, the maximum daily dose limit for the geriatric population.

Warfarin is considered a high-risk medication and drug interactions with warfarin are well known in the medical community. This resident is taking several herbal and dietary supplements that can affect the anticoagulative effects of warfarin. A possible drug interaction that may decrease the effectiveness of warfarin is reported with ubiquinol.[34] Herbal supplements reported to increase the anticoagulation of warfarin include resveratrol, pycnogenol and curcumin.[35–37] Careful monitoring for bruising and bleeding and obtaining periodic laboratory tests, including PT/INR and complete blood cell count, may be indicated.

MEDICATION REGIMEN REVIEWS FOR STAYS UNDER 30 DAYS AND CHANGES IN CONDITION

A CMS clarification letter to state survey agency directors notes the need for pharmacist medication reviews when a resident experiences a change in condition and/or for residents admitted for less than 30 days.[38] The pharmacist may need to conduct the medication review more frequently than the usual monthly review for LTC patients. According to the letter, facility procedures are expected to address the need for a medication regimen review, how it will be communicated to the provider, the expectations of the provider's response and follow-up, and the location of the documentation of review.

Because of the frequency of required medication regimen review, the consultant pharmacist visits the facility more frequently or uses the technology that is available from each facility. Off-site medication regimen reviews can be accomplished by access to computerized chart records through EHR systems or by access to secure faxes of patient information, including physician order sheets, MARs, laboratory reports, and clinical notes.

Case study 3 in **Box 4** demonstrates that drug interactions, the use of psychotropic medications, dosage formulations, and potential adverse events can be minimized prior to administration of these medications.

A drug interaction is noted in this case. For example, since 2011, the US Food and Drug Administration declared that the dose of simvastatin should be limited to 20 mg when it is coadministered with amiodarone.[39] The limitation of the dose was indicated due to the increased risk of myopathy at doses above 20 mg per day. The simvastatin (Zocor) drug label was revised to reflect the change.[40] The patient's falls may be attributed to the high dose of simvastatin due to muscle pain.

The use of psychotropic agents needs to be reviewed and monitored. As-needed orders were written for both quetiapine and alprazolam. The use of as-needed psychoactive medications must be closely scrutinized because the use of as-needed psychotropics can be considered a form of chemical restraint. The Omnibus Budget Reconciliation Act of 1987 limited the use of psychotropic medications in residents of LTC facilities; therefore, documentation of necessity and periodic trials of medication withdrawal should be attempted.[41] The questions to be addressed about these

---

Box 4
Case study 3

AA is a 78-year-old woman (no known drug allergies) who was admitted from the hospital with a diagnosis of metabolic encephalopathy, congestive heart failure, atrial fibrillation, coronary artery disease, dementia, pleural effusion, hypertension, hypothyroid, and falls.

Medications

Amiodarone, 200 mg daily

Aspirin enteric coated, 81 mg daily

Ferrous sulfate, 325 mg daily

Furosemide, 40 mg daily

Levothryoxine, 112 μg daily

Spironolactone, 50 mg q12 h

Multivitamin, 1 tablet daily

Alprazolam, 0.25 mg bid prn anxiety

Quetiapine, 25 mg q12 h prn agitation

Metoprolol succinate, 50 mg hs

Simvastatin, 80 mg daily

Potassium chloride, 20 mEq hs

Docusate, 100 mg bid

Mirabegron (Mybetriq), 50 mg hs

Lisinopril, 5 mg daily

two psychotropic orders are the duration of the need for as-needed orders, clarification of the quetiapine order to determine if it was written an as-needed order or intended as a routine order, the true indication for these behavioral modifying medications, and the attempts of nonpharmacological interventions to manage behaviors. This patient's behaviors may be due to acute and chronic illness and to pain.

During the medication regimen review during TOC, the pharmacist should also review issues of administration. This resident may have difficulty in swallowing oral medications; therefore, dosage formulations need to be reviewed. Enteric-coated aspirin and metoprolol succinate are formulations that should not be crushed. Crushable dosage forms are available for easier administration. In addition, nursing should be reminded that levothyroxine is best administered on an empty stomach and simvastatin should be administered at bedtime.

Drug-related falls are another issue that needs to be addressed. Falls among the older population are associated with a high morbidity and mortality.[42] The risk of falls may be caused by medications, such as antihypertensive agents, diuretics, β-blockers, neuroleptics and antipsychotics, and benzodiazepines.[43] This patient has an increased risk for falls due to medications as well as chronic conditions.

FINANCIAL INCENTIVES FOR MEDICATION RECONCILIATION

Clear financial incentives are currently limited and not fully directed toward the medication reconciliation process. Star rating systems have been put in place to compare nursing homes and pharmacy benefit managers. Five star ratings are awarded for superior quality and 1 star reflects quality much below average.

Medicare uses a star rating system to measure how well Medicare Advantage Plan and Medicare Prescription Drug Plan (Part D) perform, based on the 6 priorities in the National Quality Strategy.[44] One of the priorities that pertain to TOC and medication use is promoting effective communication and coordination of care. According to the National Quality Strategy, payment for this priority should reward and incentivize providers with the improvement of communication, transparency, and efficiency for better coordinated health and health care through health information technology.[45]

The nursing home Compare Five-Star Quality Rating System was instituted to help consumers make distinctions among high-performing and low-performing nursing homes. There is 1 overall star rating for each nursing home and a separate rating for health inspections, staffing, and quality measures.[46] Six new quality measures based on Medicare claims and Minimum Data Set (MDS) data were added to Nursing Home Compare.[47] This includes the percentage of short-stay patients who have had an outpatient emergency room visit and percentage of short-stay residents who were successfully discharged to the community and did not die or were readmitted to a hospital or SNF within 30 days of discharge.

Since January 1, 2015, Medicare reimburses health care providers a fee under the American Medical Association Current Procedural Terminology code for non–face-to-face care coordination services with multiple chronic conditions. Chronic care management services directed by a physician or other qualified health care professional per calendar month can receive additional payment for health services, including medication management services. Physicians and nonphysician practitioners, certified nurse midwives, clinical nurse specialists, nurse practitioners, and physician assistants can bill for these services.[48] Direct payments to pharmacists are not included for providing coordination services.

SUMMARY

Pharmacists have an opportunity to minimize polypharmacy and associated risks with medication use in LTC and AL facilities. Increased medication safety during TOC has to be addressed by an interdisciplinary team of the facilities that includes dispensing pharmacy and consultant pharmacist participation.

Facilities should have a policy and procedure for medication reconciliation within the guidelines for policies regarding admission and discharge. A guideline of how medication reconciliation is done when a patient is admitted to a facility needs to be developed with the identification of the specific roles of the nursing staff, pharmacists physicians, and other health care team members.

Continual evaluation of the medication reconciliation process needs to presented during quality assurance and performance improvement meetings. Discussions during meetings should reiterate the existing procedures and examine any pitfalls to help modify any of the procedures.

When possible, pharmacists can assist in the development of improved electronic medication record applications. Pharmacists may be able to integrate the most current medication lists with drug information and specific recommendations for patients, especially on discharge.

Finally, pharmacists can continually train and remind the nursing staff and others of the common ADEs and errors that may occur during TOC. Being vigilant to the most common errors with high-risk medications may increase medication safety.

Medication reconciliation during TOC for elderly patients is a complex process. The failure to reconcile medications during TOC accounts for preventable adverse events, which may increase hospitalizations, morbidity, and mortality. Because of the importance of patient medication safety issues, increased resources to pharmacists and health care providers are needed to implement a successful strategy to reconcile medications across health care settings.

REFERENCES

1. Routledge PA, O'Mahony MS, Woodhouse KW. Adverse drug reactions in elderly patients. Br J Clin Pharmacol 2004;57:121–6.
2. Gray CL, Gardner C. Adverse drug events in the elderly: an ongoing problem. J Manag Care Pharm 2009;15:568–71.
3. Classen DC, Pestotnik SL, Evans RS, et al. Adverse drug events in hospitalized patients. JAMA 1997;277(4):301–6.
4. Cullen DJ, Sweitzer BJ, Bates DW, et al. Preventable adverse drug events in hospitalized patients: a comparative study of intensive care and general care units. Crit Care Med 1997;25(8):1289–97.
5. Cullen DJ, Bates DW, Small SD, et al. The incident reporting system does not detect adverse drug events: a problem for quality improvement. Jt Comm J Qual Improv 1995;21(10):541–8.
6. Bates DW, Spell N, Cullen DJ, et al. The costs of adverse drug events in hospitalized patients. JAMA 1997;277(4):307–11.
7. Cornish PL, Knowles SR, Marchesano R, et al. Unintended medication discrepancies at the time of hospital admission. Arch Intern Med 2005;165(4):424–9.
8. Beers M, Munekata M, Storrie M. The accuracy of medication histories in the hospital medical records of elderly persons. J Am Geriatr Soc 1990;38:1183–7.
9. Bates DW, Cullen DJ, Laird N, et al. Incidence of adverse drug events and potential adverse drug events. JAMA 1995;274(1):29–34.

10. Budnitz DS, Shehab N, Kegler S, et al. Medication use leading to emergency department visits for adverse drug events in older adults. Ann Intern Med 2007;147(11):755–65. Available at: http://www.ncbi.nlm.nih.gov/pubmed/18056659. Accessed June 10, 2016.

11. Budnitz DS, Lovegrove MC, Shahab N, et al. Emergency hospitalizations for adverse drug events in older Americans. N Engl J Med 2011;365(21):2002–12.

12. Centers for Disease Control and Prevention, Adults and Older Adult Adverse Drug Events. Available at: http://www.cdc.gov/medicationsafety/adult_adversedrugevents.html. Accessed June 10, 2016.

13. Rudd RA, Aleshire N, Zibbell JE, et al. Increases in drug and opioid overdose deaths – United States, 2000-2014. MMWR Morb Mortal Wkly Rep 2016;64(50): 1378–82.

14. Reconcile medications at all transition points, Institute for Healthcare Improvement. Available at: http://www.ihi.org/resources/Pages/Changes/ReconcileMedicationsatAllTransitionPoints.aspx. Accessed June 10, 2016.

15. Medications at Transitions and Clinical Handoffs (MATCH) Toolkit for Medication Reconciliation, Chapter 3. Developing change: Designing the Medication Reconciliation process, Agency of Healthcare Research and Quality, Available at: http://www.ahrq.gov/professionals/quality-patient-safety/patient-safety-resources/resources/match/match3.html. Accessed June 10, 2016.

16. The High 5s Project Standard Operating Protocol, Assuring Medication Accuracy at Transitions in Care: Medication Reconciliation, Version 3, September 2014.7–8. Available at: http://www.who.int/patientsafety/implementation/solutions/high5s/h5s-sop.pdf. Accessed June 10, 2016.

17. Improving Transitions of Care, The Vision of the National Transitions of Care Coalition, Policy Paper. 2008. Available at: www.ntocc.org/Portals/0/PDF/Resources/PolicyPaper.pdf. Accessed June 10, 2016.

18. The Joint Commission, Transitions of Care: The need for collaboration across entire care continuum, Hot Topics in Health Care, Issue 2, Transitions of Care: The need for collaboration across entire care continuum. Available at: https://www.jointcommission.org/assets/1/6/TOC_Hot_Topics.pdf. Accessed June 10, 2016.

19. The Joint Commission, 2016 Long Term Care Medicare/Medicaid Certification-based option, National Patient Safety Goals. Available at: https://www.jointcommission.org/assets/1/6/2016_NPSG_LT2_ER.pdf. Accessed June 10, 2016.

20. Snow V, Beck D, Budnitz T, et al. Transitions of care Consensus policy statement: American College of Physicians, Society of General Internal Medicine, Society of Hospital Medicine, American Geriatrics Society, American College of Emergency Physicians, and Society for Academic Emergency Medicine. J Hosp Med 2009;4: 364–70.

21. American Society of Health Systems Pharmacists, Transitions of Care Resource Center. Available at: http://www.ashp.org/menu/practicepolicy/resourcecenters/transitions-of-care. Accessed June 11, 2016.

22. American Pharmacists Association, Transition of Care SIG. Available at: http://www.pharmacist.com/transitions-care-sig. Accessed June 11, 2016.

23. American Geriatrics Society, Sections and Special interest groups. Available at: http://www.americangeriatrics.org/about_us/who_we_are/sections__special_interest_groups/. Accessed June 11, 2016.

24. Federal Register/vol.80. No. 136/Thursday, July 16, 2015/Proposed Rules. Available at: https://www.federalregister.gov/articles/2015/07/16/2015-17207/medicare-and-medicaid-programs-reform-of-requirements-for-long-term-care-facilities#h-19. Accessed June 11, 2016.

25. New Jersey Universal Transfer Form. Available at: http://web.doh.state.nj.us/apps2/documents/ad/hcab_hfel7_0610.pdf. Accessed June 12, 2016.

26. Agency for Healthcare Research and Quality, Medications at Transitions and Clinical Handoffs (MATCH) Toolkit for Medication Reconciliation, Chapter 2. Figure 1: Medication Reconciliation upon Admission: High-level Process Map before redesign, revised August 2012. Available at: https://www.ahrq.gov/professionals/quality-patient-safety/patient-safety-resources/resources/match/match2.html. Accessed June 12, 2016

27. Electronic Health Record Adoption in (2014 update), American Health Information Management Association. Available at: http://library.ahima.org/doc?oid=107519#.V18GHVfPQoo. Accessed June 13, 2016.

28. Abramson E, Edwards A, Silver M, et al, HITE Investigators. Trending health information technology adoption among New York nursing homes. Am J Manag Care 2014;20(11 Spec No. 17):eSP53–9. Available at: http://www.ajmc.com/journals/issue/2014/2014-11-vol20-sp/trending-health-information-technology-adoption-among-new-york-nursing-homes. Accessed June 13, 2016.

29. Clemens S, Mileski M, Alaytsev V, et al. Adoption factors associated with electronic health record among long-term care facilities: a systematic review. BMJ Open 2015;5(1):e006615. Available at: http://www.ncbi.nlm.nih.gov/pmc/articles/PMC4316426/pdf/bmjopen-2014-006615.pdf. Accessed June 13, 2016.

30. What is subacute care? McKnight's. Available at: http://www.mcknights.com/industry-faq/what-is-subacute-care/article/104134/. Accessed June 13, 2016.

31. Weaver FM, Guihan M, Hynes D, et al. Prevalence of subacute patients in acute care: results of a study of VA hospitals. J Med Syst 1998;22(3):161–72.

32. Highlights of Prescribing Information, Exelon Patch, Dosage and administration. Available at: https://www.pharma.us.novartis.com/sites/www.pharma.us.novartis.com/files/exelonpatch.pdf. Accessed June 13, 2016.

33. Saljoughian M, Opioids: Allergy vs. Pseudoallergy, US Pharmacist, July 20, 2006; 7: HS-5-HS-9. Available at: https://www.uspharmacist.com/article/opioids-allergy-vs-pseudoallergy. Accessed June 13, 2016.

34. Possible interaction with Coenzyme Q10, University of Maryland Medical Center. Available at: http://umm.edu/health/medical/altmed/supplement-interaction/possible-interactions-with-coenzyme-q10. Accessed June 13, 2016.

35. Resveratrol, Oregon State University, Linus Pauling Institute, Micronutrient Information Center, 2016. Available at: http://lpi.oregonstate.edu/mic/dietary-factors/phytochemicals/resveratrol. Accessed June 13, 2016.

36. Pycnogenol, MedlinePlus, U.S. National Library of Medicine. Available at: https://www.nlm.nih.gov/medlineplus/druginfo/natural/1019.html. Accessed June 13, 2016.

37. Possible interaction with turmeric (or curcumin), University of Maryland Medical Center. Available at: http://umm.edu/health/medical/altmed/herb-interaction/possible-interactions-with-turmeric. Accessed June 13, 2016.

38. Nursing Homes- Clarification of Guidance related to Medication Errors and Pharmacy Services, Memorandum from the Director Survey and Certification Group to State Survey Agency Directors, Centers for Clinical Standards and Quality/Survey & Certification Group, November 2, 2012. Available at: https://www.cms.gov/Medicare/Provider-Enrollment-and-Certification/SurveyCertificationGenInfo/Downloads/Survey-and-Cert-Letter-13-02.pdf. Accessed June 13, 2016.

39. FDA Drug Safety Communication: Revised dose limitation for Zocor (simvastatin) when taken with amiodarone, US Food and Drug Administration. 2011. Available

at: http://www.fda.gov/Drugs/DrugSafety/ucm283137.htm. Accessed June 13, 2016.

40. Zocor (simvastatin) Tablets, Highlights of Prescribing Information, Reference ID:3695644. Available at: http://www.accessdata.fda.gov/drugsatfda_docs/label/2015/019766s093lbl.pdf. Accessed June 13, 2016.

41. Omnibus Budget Reconciliation Act of 1987, Public Law 100-203-Dec 22, 1987, 100th Congress. Available at: https://www.gpo.gov/fdsys/pkg/STATUTE-101/pdf/STATUTE-101-Pg1330.pdf. Accessed June 13, 2016.

42. Kannus P, Parkkari J, Koskinen S, et al. Fall-induced injuries and deaths among older adults. JAMA 1999;281:1895–9. Available at: http://jamanetwork.com/journals/jama/fullarticle/190071. Accessed June 14, 2016.

43. Woolcott J, Richardson K, Wiens M, et al. Meta-analysis of the impact of 9 medication classes on falls in elderly persons. Arch Intern Med 2009;169:1952–60. Availabe at: http://jamanetwork.com/journals/jamainternalmedicine/fullarticle/485251. Accessed June 14, 2016.

44. Department of Health and Human Services, Centers for Medicare & Medicaid Services, Letter for Request for Comments: Enhancements to the Star Ratings for 2017 and Beyond. 2015. Available at: https://www.cms.gov/Medicare/Prescription-Drug-Coverage/PrescriptionDrugCovGenIn/Downloads/2017-Star-Ratings-Request-for-Comments.pdf. Accessed June 15, 2016.

45. Payment. Available at: http://www.americangeriatrics.org/health_care_professionals/practice_management/payment_coding/. Accessed June 15, 2016.

46. Department of Health and Human Services, Centers for Medicare and Medicaid Services, Five-star Quality Rating System. Available at: https://www.cms.gov/medicare/provider-enrollment-and-certification/certificationandcomplianc/fsqrs.htm. Accessed February 7, 2017

47. Department of Health and Human Services, Centers for Medicare and Medicaid services, Press releases: CMS adds new quality measures to nursing home compare. Available at: https://www.cms.gov/newsroom/mediareleasedatabase/press-releases/2016-press-releases-items/2016-04-27.html. Accessed February 7, 2017.

48. Department of Health and Human Services, Centers for Medicare and Medicaid services, Chronic Care Management Services. Available at: https://www.cms.gov/Outreach-and-Education/Medicare-Learning-Network-MLN/MLNProducts/Downloads/ChronicCareManagement.pdf. Accessed February 7, 2017.

Can Managed Care Manage Polypharmacy?

Richard G. Stefanacci, DO, MGH, MBA, CMD[a,b,*], Taha Khan, PharmD, RPh[a]

KEYWORDS

- Polypharmacy • Managed care • Geriatrics • Beers criteria • Adherence
- Accountable Care Organizations (ACO) • Medicare Advantage Plans (MA-PD)

KEY POINTS

- Polypharmacy is the taking of multiple medications by a patient in whom the benefits are exceeded by the clinical and/or financial costs, resulting in negative or unrealized beneficial outcomes.
- Some of the common causes of polypharmacy include inappropriate application of clinical guidelines to treat multiple chronic conditions, unrecognized drug adverse events, inappropriate self-management, and the lack of patient-centered care from polyproviders, especially across care transitions.
- Managed care systems in a position to treat polypharmacy include not only traditional managed care organizations (health maintenance organizations , Medicare Advantage Plans) but newer organizations such accountable care organizations, providers involved in bundled payments and integrated delivery systems.
- Effective reduction in polypharmacy requires coordinated efforts across all key stakeholders, including prescribers, nurses, and pharmacists, and managed care is in an ideal position to provide direction and motivation; in addition to involving many stakeholders, efforts to reduce polypharmacy can occur at several points along the patient journey.
- With regard to whether managed care can manage polypharmacy, the answer is not only yes but that managed care must and can successfully treat the growing problem of polypharmacy that affects older adults and the health care system.

Polypharmacy by definition is a term used to describe multiple drug use by patients; typically, more than 4 chronic medications.[1] Under this definition, polypharmacy in many cases is appropriate. However, in practice polypharmacy has come to mean the inappropriate use of multiple medications. Polypharmacy can occur as a result of a range of situations, including the excessive application of clinical guidelines, lack of coordination among multiple prescribers, treating adverse drug events (ADEs), misaligned medications across transitions of care, patient self-treatment, and inappropriate overtreatment. The reason that polypharmacy is a problem is that

[a] The Access Group, 400 Connell Drive, Berkeley Heights, NJ 07922, USA; [b] Thomas Jefferson University, College of Population Health, 901 Walnut Street, Philadelphia, PA 19107, USA
* Corresponding author. The Access Group, 400 Connell Drive, Berkeley Heights, NJ 07922.
E-mail address: Richard.Stefanacci@jefferson.edu

Clin Geriatr Med 33 (2017) 241–255
http://dx.doi.org/10.1016/j.cger.2017.01.005
0749-0690/17/© 2017 Elsevier Inc. All rights reserved.

it often represents a situation in which the benefits of a specific medication at the dose and frequency that an individual patient is taking are outweighed by the costs. These costs can be financial; however, they may place a greater burden when they lead to unrealized benefits or adverse clinical affects.

Polypharmacy is the taking of multiple medications by a patient in which the benefits are exceeded by the clinical and/or financial costs, resulting in negative or unrealized beneficial outcomes.

The phenomenon of polypharmacy is especially prevalent among the elderly because increasing age puts adults at higher risk for multiple chronic illnesses, many of which require drug therapy. If all of the available clinical practice guidelines for older adults, such as those for management of high cholesterol levels, hypertension, diabetes, cognitive decline, and osteoporosis, were to be applied it could easily create a polypharmacy situation. The application of all of these guidelines is fast becoming a requirement for value-based payment models such as the Physician Quality Reporting System,[2] in addition to being included as components of the Welcome to Medicare and Annual Wellness Examination.[3] This process also applies in skilled nursing facilities (SNFs), in which identification of many conditions that call for treatment is a part of the minimum data set (MDS) in such sections as C for Cognition and D for Mood, both of which could lead to the use of medications under clinical guidelines that may result in polypharmacy, as noted earlier.

Polypharmacy may also result from treating adverse drug events (ADEs). For example, the most common chronic disease in the United States, osteoarthritis, affects 40 million people, most being older adults. Chronic stiffness and pain from arthritis have an impact on function, prompting the routine use of nonsteroidal antiinflammatory drugs (NSAIDs) and aspirin products. Long-term use of NSAIDs lowers the prostaglandin level in the gastrointestinal (GI) tract, which may result in esophagitis, peptic ulcerations, GI hemorrhage, and GI perforation. In older adults, treatment with histamine-2-receptor blockers or proton pump inhibitors to relieve the adverse effects of aspirin or other NSAIDs may cause additional side effects, such as confusion and mental status changes, in turn requiring more treatment. This example shows how easily adverse events occur and escalate in older patients. ADEs account for 30% of hospital admissions for persons aged 65 years and older; approximately 106,000 deaths are attributed to medication problems. Between 15% and 65% of these events are preventable[4] by avoiding potentially inappropriate medications, effective communication, and patient education.[5] When a particular medication regimen is unsuccessful, the health care provider typically prescribes another drug, which is referred to as the prescribing cascade. Dr Jerry Gurwitz, a noted geriatrician, added the caveat that "Any symptom in an elderly patient should be considered a drug side effect until proven otherwise," although his wife, Leslie Fine, a pharmacist, is thought to have first described this approach.[6]

Polypharmacy may also be attributed to patients' self-management directly through use of over-the-counter (OTC) medications, through the reuse of previously ordered medications, or through indiscriminate use from a stockpile of previously discontinued medications, primarily because of the high cost of prescription drugs. Adults may be sharing medications or may have received medications from others who thought that the drug that helped them would help their relative or friend as well. These situations are ripe for polypharmacy causing negative outcomes.

Existence of so-called polyproviders is another key driver for polypharmacy. Many older adults see multiple specialists in a variety of care settings for various acute and chronic diseases. Medications prescribed without the provider carefully reviewing the patient's other medications can lead to drug duplication and complications. Without a primary care provider overseeing the care of the older adult, adverse drug reactions are sure to occur. Providers who are not astute in the principles of safe geriatric prescribing practices may create avoidable side effects and complications. Also, medications ordered by a hospitalist for an acute stay may be appropriate in that setting but may not be needed in the outpatient setting, requiring medication reconciliation to ensure a safe and effective outpatient regimen. The current siloed prescribing practices in the hospital are being replaced by a process in which the hospital stay is used to facilitate a long-term outpatient medication plan rather than one that requires a transition and medication reconciliation. In this patient-centered approach, patients leave with an appropriate outpatient plan that takes into account their personal situations regarding treatment priorities, attitudes regarding medication, and medication access issues which could make a plan difficult to follow. Based on this approach, prescribing moves from a provider-specific/site-specific model to a patient-centered model. **Box 1** provides a summary of the common causes of polypharmacy.

Why Managed Care Should Be Used to Manage Polypharmacy

Polypharmacy contributes to health care costs for both the patient and the health care system; one study found that polypharmacy may lead to an increase of ~30% in direct medical costs, driven by increased incidence of outpatient visits and hospitalizations.[7] In a population-based study, outpatients taking 5 or more medications had an 88% increased risk of experiencing an ADE compared with those who were taking fewer medications, whereas, in nursing home residents, rates of ADEs have been noted to be twice as high in patients taking 9 or more medications compared with those taking fewer. In addition,[8] a study evaluating unplanned hospitalizations in older veterans found that patients taking more than 5 medications was almost 4 times as likely to be hospitalized because of an ADE.[8]

Polypharmacy has also been associated with functional decline in older patients, with one study showing that increased prescription medication use was associated with diminished ability to perform instrumental activities of daily living and decreased physical functioning.[8] A prospective cohort of approximately 300 older adults found that patients taking 10 or more medications had diminished functional capacity and trouble performing daily tasks.[9]

In an era in which reimbursement and financial incentives are shifting to value-based metrics rather than volume-based parameters, payers and providers are increasingly held accountable for clinical and economic outcomes through existing quality metrics and value-based payments. The burden of taking multiple medications has been

---

Box 1
Common causes of polypharmacy

- Inappropriate application of clinical guidelines to treat multiple chronic conditions
- Prescribing cascade
- Inappropriate self-management
- Lack of patient-centered care from polyproviders, especially across care transitions

associated with greater health care costs and an increased risk of ADEs, drug interactions, medication nonadherence, reduced functional capacity, and multiple geriatric syndromes.[9] Patient safety and error reduction are essential goals for health care organizations. In a consensus report on patient safety, the National Quality Forum outlined a set of best practices addressing all stakeholders across the patient care continuum to help align processes and practices.[10] Although most goals have been hospital based, managed care organizations are in a unique position to incorporate this area into their quality programs by giving support and providing incentives for areas that have been found to be valuable based on a review of evidence.

Studies have clearly validated multidisciplinary efforts, with an emphasis on pharmacists' services, in reducing polypharmacy and improving medication management, resulting in positive patient-oriented health outcomes.[9,11] One study assessed 2 interventions, 1 year apart, in high-risk patients (defined as those who were using medication across 5 categories of high-risk drug combinations). The intervention program consisted of clinical pharmacists performing drug therapy reviews, educating physicians and patients about drug safety and polypharmacy, and working with physicians and patients to correct polypharmacy problems. After the first intervention, overall rates of polypharmacy events decreased from 29 per 1000 to 9.43 per 1000 (67.5% reduction), and number of prescriptions per number per month went from 4.6 to 2.2.[12] Six months after the second intervention, the overall rate of polypharmacy was reduced from 27.99 per 1000 to 17.07 per 1000 (39% reduction),[12] so there clearly is a benefit to reducing these many issues associated with polypharmacy, but the question of how best to attack this problem, and in whom, remains.

What Is Managed Care?

With a firm understanding of what polypharmacy is and why it should be managed, the next question is whether managed care can fix polypharmacy. However, first it is necessary to understand how managed care is defined, because the definition has evolved. In its most basic form, managed care is an approach that is intended to optimize the delivery of health care services and patient care within the limitations of scarce resources.[13] It was the predominant structure for employer-based and publicly funded health care benefit plans, and is offered and administered by managed care organizations (MCOs) (**Box 2**). Select additional stakeholders within the managed care model include employers, government purchasers (Medicare, Medicaid), consumers/individual members, regulators/policy makers, clinical and professional providers, and institutional providers.[14] The assertions of an effective managed care system include alignment across all stakeholders to support the diverse needs of the enrolled population, develop business strategies that do not negatively affect the success of other types of stakeholders, share information and performance measures, be held accountable for results, and support the long-term

---

Box 2
Managed care systems

Managed care systems include:

- Traditional MCOs (health maintenance organizations, Medicare Advantage Plans)
- Accountable care organizations
- Providers involved in bundled payments
- Integrated delivery systems

needs of the entire managed care population: managing health and maintaining wellness. Despite the identification of the objectives of an effective managed care model, stakeholders have historically focused on their immediate concerns without due focus on the bigger picture, which has led to misaligned priorities and fragmented care delivery.

The advent of the Affordable Care Act (ACA) has led to a shift from fee for service to value-based payments, which has caused the creation of a variety of managed care vehicles. One of those vehicles is the Accountable Care Organization (ACO), defined as a group of doctors, hospitals, or other providers who work together to deliver coordinated care to Medicare patients.[15] ACO providers are incentivized through the Shared Savings Program and bundled payments, in which providers are paid a capitated amount based on the number of patients they care for, not the number of visits a patient makes. In this way, providers assume more risk for their patients' health but also have the opportunity to increase earnings if patients are healthy and cost less to care for because of high-quality care and better outcomes.[16] The patient-centered medical home (alternatively defined as primary care medical home [PCMH]) is another value-based care model that involves a health care delivery concept that provides an alternate understanding of how primary care is organized and delivered.[17] Although not a new concept, PCMH was brought into prominence in the US health care scene after the ACA, which subscribes greater provisions and investments to the primary care model to enhance prevention and wellness and care coordination.[18] Other models included bundled payments in which providers are responsible for a range of services, including pharmaceuticals, for a defined episode of care. These models include such episodes as cancer care in which the potential for polypharmacy is especially high because of all the issues mentioned earlier, such as polyproviders, self-medication, and ADEs. What is clear from the evolution of these new delivery models and growth of integrated delivery systems is that managed care exists in most care settings rather than being isolated to MCOs or HMOs.

What Are the Key Opportunities for Managed Care to Manage Polypharmacy?

In a truly integrated health care model, each provider interaction or touch point can be considered an opportunity to manage polypharmacy. From the primary care visit to hospital discharge to pharmacy visit, each of these are prime opportunities for health care providers to conduct drug use reviews and perform targeted interventions to address inappropriate pharmacotherapy. However, given the current practice in health care, restrictions in time, resources, or training often limit the implementation of medication management across the care continuum; managed care is in an optimal position to implement checkpoints along the patient journey while using the services of the most appropriately trained personnel.

Medication management begins with determination of the right treatment of new symptoms or issues. This approach does not always mean the introduction of a new medication, but it may warrant a dose optimization of the current medication, discontinuation of therapy, or starting nonpharmacologic treatment.[19] A new medication does not always come from a prescription, because, as previously mentioned many older adults self-medicate with OTC medications.[19] Often, these OTCs are taken without the knowledge of physicians or nursing staff, and can have interactions with existing or new prescription medications, or may mask an issue that requires provider attention. To prevent such scenarios, it is imperative for managed care to appropriately educate prescribers on the dangers of polypharmacy and how to prevent polypharmacy-related complications.

Transitions of care scenarios are highly prone to medication errors, and thus are prime opportunities for providers to prevent inappropriate polypharmacy. Recent hospitalization is often cited in the literature as a risk for polypharmacy, and may result in negative outcomes related to changes in drug therapy in the course of acute treatment in the facility.[20] Providers such as transition of care pharmacists or nurses can help reconcile medications on discharge from hospital or SNF. Evaluation of a patient's medication regimen and education of the patient and caregiver on discharge from the facility are likely to reduce duplicate therapy, inappropriate prescribing, and unnecessary medications.[20]

In addition, MCOs are ideally positioned within the health care system, which provides them with a clear view of the patient's journey from various stages of care. Having access to claims data allows health plans to analyze and identify gaps in care, and subsequently implement strategies or push communications to various providers to align objectives and improve outcomes. Pharmacist-led interventions are a prime example of how MCOs can help reduce polypharmacy; pursuant to Centers for Medicare & Medicaid Services requirements, health plans with Medicare beneficiaries who take 5 or more chronic medications must be offered medication therapy management (MTM) services by a pharmacist. The service is composed of a comprehensive medication review, in which a pharmacist carefully evaluates the need for each medication, duplication in therapy, as well as the appropriateness of each medication. Subsequently, the pharmacist conducts telephonic counseling to understand whether the patient is having ADEs or has issues with adherence. If issues are identified, the pharmacist then contacts the prescriber to advise on inappropriate medication therapy and recommend appropriate changes. Studies have shown that pharmacist-led interventions improve medication adherence, which can lead to better clinical outcomes, even for older patients on appropriate polypharmacy.[11]

In addition, managed care can provide assistive devices to reduce nonadherence issues. These devices can include compliance packaging of medications or mechanical dispensing devices that can not only alert patients when to take their medications but can also manage the timing of as-needed medications. The most sophisticated medication management devices also allow programming by prescribers or pharmacists following prescriber orders such that changes in medication regimens do not have to rely solely on patient memory to be followed. Provision of these assistive devices through managed care can assist greatly in reducing nonadherence and related polypharmacy issues.

Managed Care's Role in Managing Polypharmacy

Effective reduction in polypharmacy requires coordinated efforts across all key stakeholders, including prescribers, nurses, and pharmacists, for which managed care is in an ideal position to provide direction and motivation. In addition to involving many stakeholders, efforts to reduce polypharmacy can occur at several points along the patient journey, as described in **Table 1**.

At the start of the patient journey, appropriate benefit design can direct patients and prescribers to more appropriate medication use. However, most formularies are based on cost of medications rather than clinical appropriateness. This situation can be understood by considering the number of Beers criteria medications on plan formularies, many of which are generically available medications.

Beyond formulary design, preauthorization reviews and step therapy can be valuable in reducing polypharmacy, especially because step therapy is designed to help identify contraindications.[21] In addition, enforcing quantity limits can reduce the risk

Table 1
Managed care impact points to treat polypharmacy

	Patient	Prescriber	Pharmacist
Previsit	Benefit design: understanding coverage of pharmaceuticals through the pharmacy benefit can help patients and providers select appropriate therapy that is cost-effective and medically necessary Education on appropriate care (Rx and OTC medications)	Promote use of previsit screening/assessment	Drug use review through the patient medication list
Care (hospital, SNF, office)	Education on adherence to prescribed medications	Education on assuring right medication, including clinical pathway development and enforcement Incentives such as quality and outcomes measures to promote appropriate medication Use of motivational interviewing techniques to understand patient needs and concerns	Pharmacists as part of care team to promote more appropriate medication use
Pharmacy	MTM session with pharmacist to ensure appropriate pharmacotherapy	Understanding of drug formulary coverage to support minimum OOP cost for patient and appropriate pharmacotherapy	Education to ensure appropriate use and limit inappropriate OTC use Provider outreach to communicate duplicate or inappropriate therapy
Home	Patient and caregiver education to support adherence	Disease management programs, including nurse/case managers	MTM, including comprehensive and targeted drug review Adherence support
Follow-up visit	Patient and caregiver education to support adherence	Data analysis input on such issues as life expectancy for identification of opportunities for deprescribing when costs (clinical and financial) outweigh benefits of a medication	Ongoing MTM efforts to ensure patient understanding of medication therapy

Abbreviations: OOP, out of pocket; Rx, prescription drug.

of leftover medications and also encourage the patient to have face-to-face time with the prescriber in order to appropriately continue therapy, which may provide another opportunity to review medications.[22,23]

Even before a patient receives care, managed care can encourage patient engagement through strategies such as shared decision making and provide education on appropriate use of medications, including OTCs. This approach can help empower patients to ask the right questions to prescribers. Although the patients are given more power and participation in their health care decisions, there is an additional layer of responsibility and expectation that the patients will take measures to understand their disease and treatment in order to make informed choices.

MCOs can provide education and incentives to prescribers for the promotion of appropriate use of medications; additionally, information from claims databases and other sources can assist prescribers in identifying opportunities for medication management improvement. Reducing polypharmacy begins with the determination of the right treatment of new symptoms and issues. This approach does not always translate to the introduction of a new medication, but it can be addressed by reducing a dose of the current medication. Medication appropriateness can be assessed using the Medication Appropriate Index, which asks questions such as:

1. Is there an indication for the medication?
2. Is the dosage correct/
3. Are the directions correct? Are they practical and easy to understand?
4. Are there clinically significant drug-drug interactions?
5. Is the duration of therapy acceptable?
6. Is there unnecessary duplication with other medications?
7. Do the benefits of a specific medication outweigh the costs?

The need for the practice described earlier was shown in recently published research (http://archinte.jamanetwork.com/article.aspx?articleid=2466632). Sussman and colleagues[24] found that, among older patients whose treatment resulted in extremely low levels of hemoglobin A1c (HbA_{1c}) or blood pressure (BP), 27% or fewer underwent deintensification, representing a lost opportunity to reduce overtreatment. Further, low HbA_{1c} levels, BP values, or life expectancy had little association with deintensification events. The investigators recommended that practice guidelines and performance measures should place more focus on reducing overtreatment through deintensification.

The Beers criteria are a consensus-based system listing potentially inappropriate medications for use in older adults and guidelines for safe prescribing practices. This extensive list of medication guidelines was created by a consensus panel of nationally recognized experts in geriatrics and updated in 2015 (American Geriatrics Society [AGS] 2015); exclusion of the Beers criteria medication on a managed care formulary can reduce polypharmacy. In addition to the Beers criteria, an additional opportunity to improve outcomes and reduce polypharmacy may lie in the Choosing Wisely initiative.[25] In response to the challenge of improving health care, national organizations representing medical specialists have asked their members to choose wisely through the identification of opportunities for care improvement in their fields. The resulting list, called Things Providers and Patients Should Question, is meant to promote discussion about the need, or lack thereof, for many frequently used treatments that produce polypharmacy.

The American Medical Directors Association (AMDA) – The Society for Post-Acute and Long-Term Care Medicine identified 5 critical areas for management of pharmacotherapy in older adults (>55 years of age),[26] whereas the AGS developed 10 areas.[27]

Focusing on these 15 areas can help identify 5 common themes that can guide prescribers to improve outcomes:

1. Dementia and behavioral and psychological symptoms of dementia (BPSD)
2. Screening and medication management
3. Antibiotic use
4. Diabetes management
5. Nutritional management

These critical areas come from extensive work done by both AMDA and AGS and are refined here with a special focus on the care of older adults. Choosing Wisely starts and often ends with a wise prescriber, which can occur through education provided from an MCO. This process can occur through inclusion of these learnings within a clinical pathway that can be enforced through formulary access as well as a pay-for-performance system in which performance is based on pathway adherence and outcomes. An examination of these areas highlights specific clinical practices that managed care can provide to reduce unnecessary and costly polypharmacy.

Dementia and behavioral and psychological symptoms of dementia

A starting point is the management of dementia and BPSD, because perhaps nothing is more critical given the increasing prevalence of dementia. Several of the AMDA and AGS Choosing Wisely directives are focused in this area, including appropriate management of dementia through avoiding cholinesterase inhibitors for dementia without periodic assessment for perceived cognitive benefits and adverse GI effects. In randomized controlled trials, some patients with mild-to-moderate and moderate-to-severe Alzheimer disease achieve modest benefits in delaying cognitive and functional decline and decreasing neuropsychiatric symptoms. The impacts of cholinesterase inhibitors on institutionalization, quality of life, and caregiver burden are less well established. Clinicians, caregivers, and patients should discuss cognitive, functional, and behavioral goals of treatment before beginning a trial of cholinesterase inhibitors. Advance care planning, patient and caregiver education about dementia, diet and exercise, and nonpharmacologic approaches to behavioral issues are integral to the care of patients with dementia, and should be included in the treatment plan in addition to any consideration of a trial of cholinesterase inhibitors. If goals of treatment are not attained after a reasonable trial (eg, 12 weeks), then consider discontinuing the medication. Benefits beyond a year have not been investigated and the risks and benefits of long-term therapy have not been well established, resulting in a need for ongoing assessment.

Regarding other treatments for agitation and delirium, 2 items were raised: the use of chemical and physical restraints. Both the AGS and AMDA called out the use of antipsychotic medications because of their adverse effects and consideration as chemical restraints. Specifically, not to use antipsychotic medications for BPSD in individuals with dementia as first choice or without an assessment for an underlying cause of the behavior. People with dementia often show aggression, resistance to care, and other challenging or disruptive behaviors. In such instances, antipsychotic medicines are often prescribed, but they often provide limited benefit and can cause serious harm, including stroke and premature death.[28,29] Use of these drugs should be limited to patients in whom nonpharmacologic measures have failed and patients who pose an imminent threat to themselves or others. Identifying and addressing causes of behavior change can make drug treatment unnecessary.

Careful differentiation of causes of the symptoms (physical or neurologic vs psychiatric, psychological) may help better define appropriate treatment options. The therapeutic goal of the use of antipsychotic medications is to treat patients who present an imminent threat of harm to self or others, or are in extreme distress, and not to treat nonspecific agitation or other forms of lesser distress. Treatment of BPSD in association with the likelihood of imminent harm to self or others includes assessing for and identifying and treating underlying causes (including pain; constipation; and environmental factors such as noise or being too cold or warm), ensuring safety, reducing distress, and supporting the patient's functioning. If treatment of other potential causes of the BPSD is unsuccessful, antipsychotic medications can be considered, taking into account their significant risks compared with potential benefits. When an antipsychotic is used for BPSD, it is advisable to obtain informed consent, which is another opportunity to reduce polypharmacy.

Screening and medication management

Consider the true benefits for each older adult before recommending a screening test or medication. Treatments are often ordered based on an overestimate of the benefits and undervaluation of the risks. This tendency includes such actions as not recommending screening for breast or colorectal cancer, or prostate cancer (with the prostate-specific antigen test) without considering life expectancy and the risks of testing, overdiagnosis, and overtreatment. Cancer screening is associated with short-term risks, including complications from testing, overdiagnosis, and treatment of tumors that would not have led to symptoms. For prostate cancer, 1055 men would need to be screened and 37 would need to be treated to avoid 1 death in 11 years. For breast and colorectal cancer, 1000 patients would need to be screened to prevent 1 death in 10 years. For patients with a life expectancy less than 10 years, screening for these 3 cancers exposes them to immediate harms with little chance of benefit.

In addition, an older adult's life expectancy should be taken into account to avoid the routine use of medications to lower lipid levels in individuals with a limited life expectancy. There is no evidence that hypercholesterolemia, or low levels of high-density lipoprotein cholesterol, is an important risk factor for all-cause mortality, coronary heart disease mortality, or hospitalization for myocardial infarction or unstable angina in persons older than 70 years. Studies show that elderly patients with the lowest cholesterol levels have the highest mortality after adjusting other risk factors. In addition, a less favorable risk/benefit ratio may be seen for patients older than 85 years, in whom benefits may be more diminished and risks from statin drugs more increased (cognitive impairment, falls, neuropathy, and muscle damage).

Antimicrobial stewardship

The Centers for Disease Control and Prevention (CDC) and others are increasingly sensitive to the overuse of antibiotics. This overuse has led to dangerous drug-resistant organisms. As a result, both the AGS and AMDA made recommendations to not use antimicrobials to treat bacteriuria in older adults unless specific urinary tract symptoms are present. Cohort studies have found no adverse outcomes for older men or women associated with asymptomatic bacteriuria.[30] Antimicrobial treatment studies for asymptomatic bacteriuria in older adults show no benefits and show increased adverse antimicrobial effects.[31] Consensus criteria have been developed to characterize the specific clinical symptoms that, when associated with bacteriuria, define urinary tract infection (UTI).

The inappropriate treatment of positive urine cultures starts with an inappropriate urine analysis; as such, it is recommended not to obtain a urine culture unless there are clear signs and symptoms that localize to the urinary tract. Chronic asymptomatic bacteriuria is frequent in long-term care settings, with prevalence as high as 50%.[32] A positive urine culture in the absence of localized UTI symptoms (ie, dysuria, frequency, urgency) is of limited value in identifying whether a patient's symptoms are caused by a UTI. Colonization (a positive bacterial culture) without signs or symptoms of a localized UTI is a common problem that contributes to the overuse of antibiotic therapy, leading to an increased risk of diarrhea, resistant organisms, and infection caused by *Clostridium difficile*.[33] An additional concern is that the finding of asymptomatic bacteriuria may lead to an erroneous assumption that a UTI is the cause of an acute change of status, hence failing to detect or delaying the more timely detection of the patient's more serious underlying problem. A patient with advanced dementia may be unable to report urinary symptoms. In this situation, it is reasonable to obtain a urine culture if there are signs of systemic infection such as fever (increase in temperature of $\geq 1.1°C$ [$2°F$] from baseline), leukocytosis, or a left shift or chills in the absence of additional symptoms (eg, new cough) to suggest an alternative source of infection. Remember that it often starts with clinicians believing a patient's change in condition and requesting a urine analysis despite there not being any signs of a urinary infection. Education and enforcement of guidelines by managed care can go a long way in ensuring appropriate antibiotic use.

Diabetes management

Diabetes management was another area in which both the AGS and AMDA found common ground. The inappropriate treatment of residents with diabetes can result in falls from hypoglycemia as well as painful, frequent finger sticks and injections from the overuse of sliding-scale insulin (SSI). As a result, it is recommended to avoid using medications to achieve HbA_{1c} level less than 7.5% in most adults age 65 years and older; moderate control is generally better. There is no evidence that using medications to achieve tight glycemic control in older adults with type 2 diabetes is beneficial. Among adults who are no elderly, except for long-term reductions in myocardial infarction and mortality with metformin, using medications to achieve glycated hemoglobin levels less than 7% is associated with harms, including higher mortality. Tight[34] control has been consistently shown to produce higher rates of hypoglycemia in older adults. Given the long time frame to achieve the theorized microvascular benefits of tight control, glycemic targets should reflect patient goals, health status, and life expectancy. Reasonable glycemic targets are 7% to 7.5% in healthy older adults with long life expectancy, 7.5% to 8% in those with moderate comorbidity and a life expectancy less than 10 years, and 8% to 9% in those with multiple morbidities and shorter life expectancy.

SSI was called out to avoid using for long-term diabetes management for individuals residing in nursing homes. SSI is a reactive way of treating hyperglycemia after it has occurred rather than preventing it. Good evidence exists that SSI is not effective in meeting the body's insulin needs.[35] Use of SSI leads to greater patient discomfort because patients' blood glucose levels are usually monitored more frequently than may be necessary and more insulin injections may be given. With SSI regimens, patients may be at risk from prolonged periods of hyperglycemia. In addition, the risk of hypoglycemia is a significant concern because insulin may be administered without regard to meal intake. Basal insulin, or basal plus rapid-acting insulin with 1 or more meals (often called basal/bolus insulin therapy), most closely mimics normal physiologic insulin production and controls blood glucose more effectively.[36] Managed care can increase awareness of inappropriate SSI with recommendations for changes to scheduled dosing or oral insulin treatments.

Nutritional support
In addition, appropriate nutritional support is often critical at the end of life. This support involves avoiding inappropriate nutritional interventions. One such intervention is percutaneous feeding tubes. It is recommended not to use percutaneous feeding tubes in individuals with advanced dementia. Instead, offer oral assisted feedings. Strong evidence exists that artificial nutrition does not prolong life or improve quality of life in patients with advanced dementia.[37] Substantial functional decline and recurrent or progressive medical illnesses may indicate that a patient who is not eating is unlikely to obtain any significant or long-term benefit from artificial nutrition. Feeding tubes are often placed after hospitalization, frequently with concerns for aspirations, and for those who are not eating. Contrary to what many people think, tube feeding does not ensure the patient's comfort or reduce suffering; it may cause fluid overload, diarrhea, abdominal pain, local complications, and less human interaction, and may increase the risk of aspiration. Assistance with oral feeding is an evidence-based approach to provide nutrition for patients with advanced dementia and feeding problems.

Also called out regarding nutritional support was avoiding the use of prescription appetite stimulants or high-calorie supplements for treatment of anorexia or cachexia in older adults; instead, optimize social supports, provide feeding assistance, and clarify patient goals and expectations. Unintentional weight loss is a common problem for medically ill or frail elderly. Although high-calorie supplements increase weight in older people, there is no evidence that they affect other important clinical outcomes, such as quality of life, mood, functional status, or survival. Use of megestrol acetate results in minimal improvements in appetite and weight gain, no improvement in quality of life or survival, and increased risk of thrombotic events, fluid retention, and death.[38] In patients who take megestrol acetate, 1 in 12 have an increase in weight and 1 in 23 die.[39] The 2012 AGS Beers criteria list megestrol acetate and cyproheptadine as medications to avoid in older adults (AGS, 2012). Systematic reviews of cannabinoids, dietary polyunsaturated fatty acids (docosahexaenoic acid [DHA] and eicosapentaenoic acid [EPA]), thalidomide, and anabolic steroids have not identified adequate evidence for the efficacy and safety of these agents for weight gain. Mirtazapine is likely to cause weight gain or increased appetite when used to treat depression, but there is little evidence to support its use to promote appetite and weight gain in the absence of depression. Overall, managed care can assist by increasing family involvement in feeding and promoting the activity of oral feeding to prevent the potential inappropriate use of a pharmacotherapy.

The 5 areas of dementia and BPSD management, screening and medication management, antibiotic use, diabetes management and nutritional management are critical to improving outcomes and reducing polypharmacy. A common thread through these Choosing Wisely initiatives is prudent use of services such that individual patient care is based on the benefits clearly exceeding the costs (clinical and financial). This balance requires thoughtful assessments to ensure that interventions are not encouraged that are not of benefit for that particular patient. In the end, managed care can play a key role in ensuring that every patient receives appropriate care and avoids polypharmacy.

Deprescribing when the costs of a medication (clinical and financial) outweigh the benefits requires that prescribers appreciate an older adult's life expectancy and goals of care, and this is critical for determination of when discontinuation of treatments is appropriate. To aid in the determination of prognosis there is a calculator available to health care providers through www.ePrognosis.org. The information on ePrognosis is intended as a rough guide to inform health care providers about possible mortality outcomes. This information can assist in making a determination when a medication such as a statin may no longer be appropriate because of a limited life expectancy. This situation is unique to older adults, because in the care of younger adults discontinuation because of limited effectiveness secondary to a shortened life expectancy is typically not an issue. By managed care providing life expectancy information for specific patients, opportunities for deprescribing can occur. In addition to managed care educating prescribers on opportunities for when deprescribing is appropriate, managed care can also provide information on how to deprescribe medications that require careful monitoring and titration to discontinue to avoid adverse events.

Pharmacists have had an important role for decades, at the pharmacy counter, preventing drug-drug interactions and identifying medication contraindications and adverse events. However, modern pharmacists practice at various sites of care; for example, these valued members of the health care team are in hospitals, offices, and SNF settings. Pharmacist-led intervention, such as MTM and telephonic counseling, has been shown to have a positive impact on reducing the number of patients' medications, and other opportunities to address polypharmacy include appropriate prescribing and medication reconciliation, especially in transitions of care, by physicians and nurses.[40] Pharmacist-led MTM programs, which include retrospective medication reviews, disease management, and targeted interventions, have shown plausible reductions in inappropriate polypharmacy among elderly patients. In a meta-analysis including 14 studies that assessed the impact of pharmacists on the reduction of polypharmacy in the elderly, pharmacist intervention in medication management and monitoring led to reduction in the number of drugs prescribed to elderly patients.[41] In addition, motivational interviewing techniques may help improve patient engagement across providers, including physicians, nurses, and pharmacists, and can lead to better understanding of disease state, medications, and lifestyle modifications (see **Table 1**).[11,42,43]

The Future of Managed Care Management of Polypharmacy

The importance of treating polypharmacy will become even more acute because of the growing population of older adults and limited resources. Opportunities for managed care to lead this effort will increase as health care continues to move from a fee-for-service to a value-based care system; all providers will operate under a form of managed care. It is within these managed care structures, such as Medicare Advantage Plans, ACOs, bundled payment providers, and integrated delivery network (IDNs), that systems will put into place processes to prevent and eliminate polypharmacy. In a value-based system, polypharmacy is a situation in which investing resources in managing care will realize sizable returns. Because these systems are charged with delivery of the triple aim of cost efficiency, delivering patient-centered quality care, and population health outcomes, this realization is only possible if polypharmacy is properly managed. With regard to the question of whether managed care can manage polypharmacy, the answer is not only yes but that managed care must and can successfully treat the growing problem of polypharmacy affecting older adults and the health care system.

REFERENCES

1. Milton J, Jackson S. Inappropriate polypharmacy: reducing the burden of multiple medication. Clin Med 2007;7:514–7.

2. Physician Quality Reporting System (PQRS). Centers for Medicare and Medicaid Services. Available at: https://www.cms.gov/Medicare/Quality-Initiatives-Patient-Assessment-Instruments/PQRS/index.html?redirect=/pqri. Accessed August 4, 2016.

3. Department of Health and Human Services. Centers for Medicare & Medicaid Services. The ABCs of the Annual Wellness Visit (AWV). Available at: https://www.cms.gov/Outreach-and-Education/Medicare-Learning-Network-MLN/MLNProducts/downloads/AWV_chart_ICN905706.pdf. Accessed August 4, 2016.
4. Shiyanbola OO, Farris KB. Concerns and beliefs about medicines and inappropriate medications: an Internet-based survey on risk factors for self-reported adverse drug events among older adults. Am J Geriatr Pharmacother 2010; 8(3):245–57.
5. Available at: https://www.ascp.com/articles/prescribing-cascade/. Accessed August 3, 2016.
6. Gurwitz J, Monane M, Monane S, et al. Polypharmacy. In: Morris JN, Lipsitz LA, Murphy K, et al, editors. Quality care in the nursing home. St. Louis (MO): Mosby Yearbook; 1997. p. 13–25.
7. Available at: http://medstopper.com/files/Polypharmacy_adverse-drug_reactions_geriatric.pdf. Accessed August 3, 2016.
8. Maher RL, Hanlon JT, Hajjar ER. Clinical consequences of polypharmacy in elderly. Expert Opin Drug Saf 2014;13(1):57–65.
9. Maher R, Hanlon J, Hajjar E. Clinical consequences of polypharmacy in elderly. Expert Opin Drug Saf 2014;13(1):1–11.
10. Available at: http://www.qualityforum.org/News_And_Resources/Press_Kits/Safe_Practices_for_Better_Healthcare.aspx. Accessed August 3, 2016.
11. Lee JK, Alshehri S, Kutbi HI, et al. Optimizing pharmacotherapy in elderly patients: the role of pharmacists. Integr Pharm Res Pract 2015;4:101–11.
12. Zarowitz BJ, Stebelsky LA, Muma BK, et al. Reduction of high-risk polypharmacy drug combinations in patients in a managed care setting. Pharmacotherapy 2005;25(11):1636–45.
13. Navarro R, Cahill J. Role of managed care in the US healthcare system. Growth of managed care [textbook]. Available at: http://www.jblearning.com/samples/0763732400/32400_CH01_Pass2.pdf. Accessed May 26, 2016.
14. Schield J, Murphy J, Bolnick H. Evaluating managed care effectiveness: a societal perspective. North Am Actuarial J 2001;5(4):1–41.
15. Available at: https://www.cms.gov/Medicare/Medicare-Fee-for-Service-Payment/ACO/index.html?redirect=/aco. Accessed August 4, 2016.
16. Accountable Care Organizations (ACO). CMS.gov [Web site]. Available at: https://www.cms.gov/Medicare/MedicareFeeforServicePayment/ACO/index.html?redirect=/ACO/. Accessed May 26, 2016.
17. Available at: https://pcmh.ahrq.gov/. Accessed August 5, 2016.
18. History: Major milestones for primary care and medical home. Patient-Centered Primary Care Collaborative [Web site]. Available at: https://www.pcpcc.org/content/history-0. Accessed May 26, 2016.
19. Stefanacci R, Haimowitz D. Medication management in assisted living. Geriatr Nurs 2015;33(4):304.e1-11.
20. Rambhade S, Chakarborty A, Shrivastava A. A survey on polypharmacy and use of inappropriate medications. Toxicol Int 2012;19(1):68–73.
21. Available at: http://www.bcbsm.com/index/health-insurance-help/faqs/plan-types/pharmacy/what-is-step-therapy.html. Accessed August 4, 2016.
22. Daughton C, Ruhoy I. Lower-dose prescribing: minimizing "side effects" of pharmaceuticals on society and the environment. Sci Total Environ 2013;443:324–37.
23. Porter M, Lee T. The strategy that will fix health care. Harvard Business Review [online] 2013 Oct. https://hbr.org/2013/10/the-strategy-that-will-fix-health-care. Accessed May 26, 2016.

24. Sussman JB, Kerr EA, Saini SD, et al. Rates of deintensification of blood pressure and glycemic medication treatment based on levels of control and life expectancy in older patients with diabetes mellitus. JAMA Intern Med 2015;175(12): 1942–9.

25. Choosing Wisely. Available at: http://www.choosingwisely.org/. Accessed August 3, 2016.

26. Choosing Wisely. Available at: http://www.choosingwisely.org/societies/amda-the-society-for-post-acute-and-long-term-care-medicine/. Accessed August 5, 2016.

27. Choosing Wisely. Available at: http://www.choosingwisely.org/societies/american-geriatrics-society/. Accessed August 5, 2016.

28. Available at: http://www.fda.gov/Drugs/DrugSafety/PostmarketDrugSafety InformationforPatientsandProviders/ucm124830.htm. Accessed August 3, 2016.

29. Maust DT, Kim HM, Seyfried LS, et al. Antipsychotics, other psychotropics, and the risk of death in patients with dementia: number needed to harm. JAMA Psychiatry 2015;72(5):438–45.

30. Rowe TA, Juthani-Mehta M. Urinary tract infection in older adults. Aging health 2013;9(5). http://dx.doi.org/10.2217/ahe.13.38.

31. Available at: https://www.healthplexus.net/files/content/2003/October/0609 bacteriuria.pdf. Accessed August 4, 2016.

32. Drinka P. Treatment of bacteriuria without urinary signs, symptoms, or systemic infectious illness (S/S/S). J Am Med Dir Assoc 2009;10(8):516–9.

33. Zabarsky TF, Sethi AK, Donskey CJ. Sustained reduction in inappropriate treatment of asymptomatic bacteriuria in a long-term care facility through an educational intervention. Am J Infect Control 2008;36(7):476–80.

34. ACCORD Study Group, Gerstein HC, Miller ME, et al. Effects of intensive glucose lowering in type 2 diabetes. N Engl J Med 2008;258(24):2545–59.

35. Hirsch IB. Sliding scale insulin—time to stop sliding. JAMA 2009;301(2):213–4.

36. Available at: http://www.diabetesselfmanagement.com/blog/use-basal-insulin/. Accessed August 5, 2016.

37. Finucane TE, Christmas C, Travis K. Tube feeding in patients with advanced dementia: a review of the evidence. JAMA 1999;282(14):1365–70.

38. Fox CB, Treadway AK, Blaszczyk AT, et al. Megestrol acetate and mirtazapine for the treatment of unplanned weight loss in the elderly. Pharmacotherapy 2009; 29(4):383–97.

39. Ruiz Garcia V, López-Briz E, Carbonell Sanchis R, et al. Megestrol acetate for treatment of anorexia-cachexia syndrome. Cochrane Database Syst Rev 2013;(3):CD004310.

40. Exploring pharmacists' role in a changing health care environment. Avalere Health. Available at: http://www.nacds.org/pdfs/comm/2014/pharmacist-role. pdf. Accessed August 5, 2016.

41. Marek KD, Antle L. Medication management of the community-dwelling older adult. In: Hughes RG, editor. Patient safety and quality: an evidence-based handbook for nurses. Rockville (MD): Agency for Healthcare Research and Quality (US); 2008. p. 1–38. Available at: https://www.ncbi.nlm.nih.gov/books/ NBK2670/. Accessed February 10, 2017.

42. Rollason V, Vogt N. Reduction of polypharmacy in the elderly: a systematic review of the role of the pharmacist. Quality-assessed reviews [Internet]. York (United Kingdom): Centre for Reviews and Dissemination (UK); 2003.

43. Sipkoff M. Put all your drugs into a bag and take it to your pharmacist. Manag Care 2006;15(2):14–6.

Medication Risk Mitigation

Coordinating and Collaborating with Health Care Systems, Universities, and Researchers to Facilitate the Design and Execution of Practice-Based Research

Kevin T. Bain, PharmD, MPH*, Calvin H. Knowlton, BPharm, MDiv, PhD,
Jacques Turgeon, BPharm, PhD

KEYWORDS

- Polypharmacy • Medication risk mitigation • Medication therapy management
- Pharmacy practice • Personalized medicine • Pharmacogenomics

KEY POINTS

- Polypharmacy is highly prevalent and a predictor of poor health outcomes in geriatric patients.
- Traditional medication risk mitigation (MRM) strategies, most notably pharmacist-provided medication therapy management services, are necessary to improve polypharmacy; however, they are not sufficient to improve therapeutic outcomes.
- Using multidrug analysis software to make intelligent predictions about complex drug interactions and pharmacogenomics (PGx) to predict which geriatric patients may respond to specific medications are examples of enhanced MRM strategies that may prove to be more effective than traditional MRM strategies.
- Advances in integrating PGx into clinical practice have been made but significant barriers remain. Widespread integration of PGx requires overcoming these barriers and a health care professional champion group, which we propose will be pharmacists.

Disclosure Statement: Tabula Rasa HealthCare, and the authors as stakeholders in Tabula Rasa HealthCare, have financial interests in the new multidrug analysis software the company has developed (Medication Risk Mitigation Matrix [Patent Pending]). This article, in parts or full, has not been submitted or presented elsewhere.
Science, Education, and Research Department, Tabula Rasa HealthCare, Inc, 228 Strawbridge Drive, Moorestown, NJ 08057, USA
* Corresponding author.
E-mail address: KBain@tabularasahealthcare.com

Clin Geriatr Med 33 (2017) 257–281
http://dx.doi.org/10.1016/j.cger.2017.01.009
0749-0690/17/© 2017 Elsevier Inc. All rights reserved.

geriatric.theclinics.com

INTRODUCTION

Medications are a fundamental component of the care of geriatric patients. Optimization of medication use for geriatric populations has become an important public health issue worldwide. Used appropriately, medications can prevent or slow the onset or worsening of many medical conditions, alleviate distressing symptoms, and improve health outcomes.[1] Too often, however, medications are not used appropriately in geriatric patients.[1–3]

Polypharmacy, defined as the use of multiple medications, is highly prevalent in geriatric populations and has been identified as the principal determinant of inappropriate medication use and medication-related problems (MRPs).[4–8] MRPs include, but are not limited to, adverse drug reactions and drug interactions (**Table 1**). The potential for adverse drug events (ADEs) and negative health outcomes with polypharmacy and MRPs in geriatric patients is well documented.[9–14] Incidence estimates suggest that nearly one in five hospital admissions is because of an ADE[11,12,15,16]; similarly, while in the hospital, close to one in five geriatric patients experiences an ADE.[17,18] Mitigating medication risk in geriatric patients is of considerable importance because ADEs are potentially preventable up to 50% of the time[19,20] and have considerable cost implications for health care systems, notwithstanding the cost and health implications for patients.

The prospect of attaining a future with better balance between caring for geriatric patients and avoiding medication-related harm is today's possibility through advanced technology and practice-based research. With the growing awareness of MRPs coupled with regulatory requirements and potential penalties, health care providers are actively strategizing to mitigate medication risk to reduce ADEs and optimize therapeutic outcomes for geriatric patients.[21] This article provides a narrative review of traditional medication risk mitigation (MRM) strategies to facilitate the design and execution of practice-based research for enhanced MRM strategies.

TRADITIONAL MEDICATION RISK MITIGATION STRATEGIES

Team-based health care for geriatric patients is gaining traction in the United States.[22] The changing landscape of geriatric care requires a clear understanding of how health care systems, organizations, and professionals can coordinate and

Table 1 Types and definitions of MRPs	
Type	**Definition**
Untreated indication	Needing a drug but not having it prescribed
Improper drug selection	Taking or receiving the wrong drug
Subtherapeutic dosage	Taking or receiving too little of the correct drug
Supratherapeutic dosage	Taking or receiving too much of the correct drug
Failure to receive drug	Not taking or receiving the drug as prescribed
Drug use without indication	Taking a drug for which there is no medically valid indication
Drug interaction	A clinically meaningful interaction involving a drug
Adverse drug reaction	An appreciably harmful or unpleasant reaction to a drug

Data from Strand LM, Morley PC, Cipolle RJ, et al. Drug-related problems: their structure and function. DICP 1990;24(11):1093–7; and Hepler CD, Strand LM. Opportunities and responsibilities in pharmaceutical care. Am J Hosp Pharm 1990;47(3):533–43.

collaborate to address unmet patient needs, provide high-quality health care, contribute to positive health outcomes, and influence health care use and costs. In this context, we examine the evolving role of pharmacists as collaborative members of health care teams, as other health care professionals and organizations within the system take on different levels of risks and forge new partnerships. Although other health care professionals have extensive education, skills, and training that make them uniquely qualified to provide clinical services for geriatric patients within team-based health care, through their focused training in pharmacodynamics, pharmacokinetics, and medication management, pharmacists are ideally qualified to mitigate medication risk.

Traditionally, pharmacists' role in health care centered around dispensing medications in accordance with a prescription and providing a final check to ensure accurate delivery of medications to patients.[22] According to the 2014 National Pharmacist Workforce Survey, pharmacists are stepping away from their traditional role and providing more direct patient care,[23] and their role continues to evolve today. As pharmacists continue to collaborate as part of geriatric patients' team of health care professionals, it is important to understand the types of services pharmacists provide, their capacity to meaningfully improve health care, and how these services can align with the changing landscape of geriatric care.[22] To focus this discussion, we identify a core pharmacist service: medication therapy management (MTM). Some health care payers, including Centers for Medicare and Medicaid Services (CMS), are playing a decisive role in leveraging and evolving pharmacist-provided MTM services. As such, pharmacists have a great opportunity to improve public health through better management of geriatric patients' medication therapy.

Traditional Medication Therapy Management

Background

As defined in a consensus definition adopted by the pharmacy profession in 2004, MTM is a distinct service or group of services that optimize therapeutic outcomes for patients.[24,25] The definition supports MTM as distinct from medication dispensing services and the routine patient counseling services provided by a pharmacist when a patient picks up a prescription medication.[25] These brief, patient counseling services usually involve education about a particular medication being dispensed (eg, administration instructions), and address the patient's questions specifically relating to that particular medication. In contrast, MTM is a patient-centered service that encompasses the assessment and evaluation of a patient's complete medication therapy (including over-the-counter medications, herbals, and supplements), rather than focusing on a particular medication, and that comprehensively addresses a patient's full range of potential or actual MRPs, rather than just addressing the patient's questions.[24,25]

Building on the consensus definition, the American Pharmacists Association and the National Association of Chain Drug Stores Foundation developed a model framework for the provision of MTM services by pharmacists. The framework is designed to empower patients to be self-advocates; enhance communication between patients and their health care team; improve collaboration among pharmacists, prescribers, and other health care professionals; and optimize medication use for improved patient outcomes.[25] This framework established core elements for all MTM services provided by pharmacists. According to the framework, the five core elements of pharmacist-provided MTM services are (1) medication therapy review, (2) personal medication record, (3) medication-related action plan, (4) intervention and/or referral, and (5) documentation and follow-up.[25]

Following passage of the Medicare Prescription Drug, Improvement, and Modernization Act (MMA) of 2003, prescription drug plans (PDPs) and Medicare Advantage PDPs were required to offer MTM programs to eligible Medicare beneficiaries, beginning in 2006. Beneficiaries who had multiple medical conditions, prescribed multiple Part D medications, and likely to exceed a certain threshold in annual costs for covered Part D medications (eg, $3138 in 2015) were considered eligible for these MTM programs. However, eligible beneficiaries in many plans initially had to opt in to MTM programs. This provision has since been changed so that eligible beneficiaries are offered to participate in MTM programs unless they opt out.

The MMA established MTM programs to ensure Part D medications are used appropriately and to reduce ADEs and optimize therapeutic outcomes for Medicare beneficiaries through improved medication use. However, criteria required to qualify Part D plans as MTM program providers were not explicitly stated in the MMA legislation. Furthermore, although the legislation did not specify how the components of MTM programs (ie, MTM services) should be delivered and by whom, pharmacists were specifically mentioned in the MMA as one of the key health care professionals that should provide MTM services. Today, pharmacists provide MTM services to a wide variety of patient populations in addition to Medicare beneficiaries.

Evidence

Over the past decade since the passage of the MMA, the evidence base for pharmacist-provided MTM services has grown markedly and spans multiple therapeutic areas (eg, cardiology, mental health) and care settings, including outpatient and inpatient settings.[22] A summary of the evidence base indicates the effectiveness of pharmacist-provided MTM services as (1) improving medication adherence, (2) improving quality of prescribing (ie, reducing inappropriate prescribing/improving appropriate prescribing), and (3) reducing certain MRPs.[1,4,14,22,26–30]

Although there is an extensive body of evidence for the effectiveness of pharmacist-provided MTM services on improving medication use, particularly among geriatric patients, there is conflicting evidence for whether these MTM services result in meaningful improvements in therapeutic outcomes. Some studies have not shown improvements in therapeutic outcomes,[1,4,27,29–33] whereas others demonstrated that pharmacist-provided MTM services improve clinical outcomes (eg, improve measures of disease status, such as blood pressure and cholesterol, and reduce hospital admissions),[28,34–41] humanistic outcomes (eg, improve patient satisfaction, improve quality of life),[42,43] and/or economic outcomes (eg, lower total health care costs, reduction in per member per month prescription costs).[21,28,33,35–38,42,44,45] Adding to the conflicting evidence, several recently published systematic reviews and meta-analyses of traditional MTM services have graded the evidence for these services as insufficient and poor quality with respect to improvement in most health outcomes.[1,4,46]

Future directions

The differences in outcomes achieved across MTM service providers has been attributed to marked variation in research study design and significant study limitations.[1,22,28,46] Differences also have been attributed to the traditional MTM model itself. Based on a third-party report to CMS,[28] reasons that the traditional MTM model fall short of its potential to enable Part D plans to consistently and demonstrably improve therapeutic outcomes include that (1) emphasis has been placed on procedural processes and metrics to meet compliance standards and satisfy CMS requirements; (2) MTM programs are not incentivized nor rewarded for performance, rather, standalone Part D plans are at risk for medication costs only and do not necessarily have an incentive to resolve MRPs to improve outcomes and reduce downstream health care costs; and (3) there is lack of consensus on appropriate Part D MTM measures that are truly outcomes-based. The result is that Part D MTM resources may be misallocated and accordingly fail to support MTM services that are likely to have the greatest effect on patient health outcomes.[47]

With the increasing complexity of medication use in the aging population, MTM is necessary to mitigate medication risk and optimize therapeutic outcomes for geriatric patients.[38] Now more than ever, as unsustainable health care costs persist in the United States, payers are focused on value. According to CMS, the current landscape is that Part D plans are delivering MTM services only at a level necessary to meet the minimal government compliance standards and these models are not well-aligned with government quality improvement and financial interests.[47] Notwithstanding the aforementioned recognized effectiveness of pharmacist-provided MTM services, the recently published systematic reviews and meta-analyses support the CMS conclusion that traditional MTM services are necessary but not sufficient.

Tools to Facilitate Traditional Medication Therapy Management

Drug interaction tools

An important MRP that frequently occurs in geriatric patients is drug-drug interactions (DDIs).[48–50] It has been estimated that the prevalence of DDIs in geriatric populations is 70% to 80%.[48,50,51] One study estimated that the probability of at least one clinically relevant DDI is 50% in geriatric patients taking five to nine medications, 81% with 10 to 14 medications, 92% with 15 to 19 medications, and 100% with 20 or more medications.[48] Furthermore, the addition of each medication to a five-drug regimen confers an approximate 12% increase in risk for potential DDIs.[48]

It is common practice for pharmacists to use drug alert software programs to detect DDIs while performing a medication therapy review as part of MTM services. In fact, most of these programs are sold by a small number of firms and have been on the market and in use in pharmacies across the country for decades. Unfortunately, traditional drug alert software programs have major shortcomings.[52–55] Foremost, these programs only display pairwise (ie, two-drug) interactions, which are difficult to extrapolate to geriatric patients with polypharmacy and using multiple potentially interacting medications simultaneously.[48,49] In clinical practice, geriatric patients may use multiple substrates of a hepatic cytochrome P-450 (CYP) enzyme or use an inhibitor and an inducer of the same CYP enzyme, rendering the prediction of the clinical relevance of these interactions difficult, especially when detected in a pairwise manner.[49] Furthermore, the high frequency of two-drug interaction alerts generated by these software programs has contributed to considerable dissatisfaction and frustration among pharmacists and other health care professionals, and reported override rates for DDI alerts consistently exceed 90%.[56–61]

In the largest and most comprehensive study of its kind, reporters from the Chicago Tribune recently tested 255 pharmacies to see how often pharmacists would dispense medications involved in dangerous DDIs without warning patients and despite the use of drug alert software programs.[62] Overall, 52% of the pharmacies dispensed the medications without warning patients of the actual or potential interactions.[62] More specifically, one of the nation's largest chain pharmacies had the lowest failure rate at 30%, yet this translated into still missing nearly one in three DDIs, including potentially fatal interactions.[62] Notwithstanding the significance of this report, disappointingly, it is not the first of its kind. In 1996, researchers determined the likelihood that pharmacists would fill prescriptions for two medications whose concomitant use was contraindicated (terfenadine and ketoconazole).[63] In this study, among the 48 pharmacies using drug alert software programs, approximately one-third of pharmacies filled the two medications.[63] Although a comprehensive review of the major software programs on the market is beyond the scope of this article, these data provide compelling evidence that currently available drug interaction tools either are insufficient in their detection of DDIs or are ignored by pharmacists; moreover, innovative tools are needed to allow DDIs to become more accurate and predictable and to provide enhanced clinical support to pharmacists for mitigating drug interactions in geriatric patients.

Medication appropriateness tools

As part of MTM services, pharmacists often use validated tools to assess prescribing appropriateness for geriatric patients. A recently published Cochrane systematic review concluded that, overall, interventions using these tools demonstrated improvements in appropriate polypharmacy among geriatric patients, based on reductions in inappropriate prescribing.[4] Commonly used validated tools as part of MTM services include the following: Medication Appropriateness Index, Beers Criteria, and Screening Tool of Older Person's Prescriptions/Screening Tool to Alert Doctors to Right Treatment Criteria.[4,19,64,65]

Despite the use of validated tools that result in reductions in inappropriate prescribing, according to the Cochrane systematic review, it remains unclear if these reductions result in clinically meaningful improvements in health outcomes (eg, reduction in hospitalizations) for geriatric patients.[4]

ENHANCED MEDICATION RISK MITIGATION STRATEGIES
Enhanced Medication Therapy Management

Background

On September 28, 2015, CMS announced an empowering new MTM model, the Part D Enhanced MTM Model, which provides financial incentives and regulatory flexibility to Part D plans to encourage meaningful innovation in MTM services.[47] CMS is conducting a test of this model in 5 of the 34 existing US Part D regions (ie, Region 7, Region 11, Region 21, Region 25, and Region 28) through the Center for Medicare and Medicaid Innovation.[47] The Part D Enhanced MTM Model is designed to test changes to the Part D program that would achieve better alignment of PDP sponsor and government financial interests (ie, reducing Part D prescription costs and reducing net Medicare expenditures), while also creating incentives for robust investment and innovation in better MTM services to reduce ADEs and optimize therapeutic outcomes and to enhance or improve patient satisfaction.[47] CMS anticipates the model will begin on January 1, 2017, and the proposed duration of the initial model test performance period is 5 years.[47] The full duration of the model test will span 7 years, because Center for Medicare and Medicaid Innovation will continue to make performance-based payments for 2 additional years after the model performance period.[47]

The components of this model differ from and replace the current Part D MTM program requirements. However, all Part D medication costs will remain "inside" the Part D plan's annual bid to CMS.[47] According to CMS, key elements of the Part D Enhanced MTM Model will include (1) significant regulatory flexibilities to allow PDP sponsors and Part D plans to design and implement more personalized and risk-stratified MTM services; (2) a direct prospective payment to PDP sponsors to support the cost of expanding MTM services that will be "outside" of a Part D plan's annual bid to CMS; and (3) a performance payment, in the form of an increased direct premium subsidy, for PDP sponsors that successfully improve outcomes and reduce Medicare

Part A and/or Part B expenditures and fulfill quality and other data reporting requirements through the model.[47]

Future directions

The regulatory flexibilities of the Part D Enhanced MTM Model permit participating PDP sponsors to risk stratify the population enrolled in their Part D plans with respect to medication-related risk and to offer different intensities and types of MTM services based on beneficiary risk level, instead of providing the same level to all targeted beneficiaries, as is the current (traditional) MTM strategy.[47] The regulatory flexibilities also allow PDP sponsors to provide beneficiary incentives and cost sharing assistance to enhance access to MTM services and ensure participation.[47] Sponsors also have the flexibility to experiment with alternative documentation (beyond the standardized Comprehensive Medication Review format) to improve beneficiary and prescriber communication and engagement.[47] CMS hopes to evaluate, if left to their own designs, whether Part D plans can identify and overcome barriers to effective MTM.

If successful, the Part D Enhanced MTM Model will result in PDP sponsors and CMS learning how to identify and implement innovative strategies to optimize medication use, improve care coordination, and strengthen system linkages between Part D plans, pharmacists, and prescribers.[47] To accomplish these goals, PDP sponsors will need to leverage the core competencies of their own organizations and of their network pharmacy providers with those of prescribers to accurately identify and effectively intervene with all beneficiaries whose issues with medication management have caused, or are likely to cause, adverse outcomes and/or significant nondrug program use and costs.[47] This new MTM model creates a potential opportunity for health care professionals (especially pharmacists), organizations, and systems to improve care and outcomes for millions of geriatric patients in the United States.

Innovative Strategies for Enhanced Medication Therapy Management

Drug interaction tools

Background Pharmacists may be better suited than other health care professionals to manage DDIs based on their extensive training in pharmacodynamics and pharmacokinetics.[48] Yet, previously mentioned data indicate that pharmacists need to be equipped with innovative DDI support tools to manage complex DDIs that commonly occur in geriatric patients with polypharmacy. Until recently, there was no simple way to make intelligent predictions about the likelihood or severity of multidrug CYP-mediated DDIs. However, CYP-specific multidrug analysis software has been developed and deployed by the authors (ie, Medication Risk Mitigation Matrix, Moorestown, NJ). The software program lists all of a patient's medications simultaneously and displays the relative affinity of each medication for each CYP enzyme to assess competitive inhibition between strong, moderate, and weak enzyme substrates.[48,51] It highlights, in a single-page color-coded matrix, all potential DDIs between not only substrates of the same CYP enzyme (ie, competitive inhibition) but also between CYP enzyme inhibitors and/or inducers (ie, noncompetitive inhibition), based on a bioequivalence standard of 30% and published pharmacokinetic data.[48] The CYP-specific multidrug analysis software also examines drug-gene interactions (DGIs), when genetic results are available, and it simultaneously analyzes an array of additional MRM factors (eg, cognitive risk, heart rhythm disorder risk) on an individual patient and population basis. Additionally, the software program allows pharmacists, and other health care professional users, to make virtual changes to a patient's medications for making optimal decisions regarding mitigating medication risk.

Evidence In a prospective comparison study, the prevalence of potential CYP-mediated DDIs detected by the multidrug analysis software program among 275 geriatric patients (mean [± standard deviation] age, 83 [8] years; range, 65–103 years) with polypharmacy was 80%,[48] which was similar to a previous study of the software program.[51] Of the 221 patients with potential CYP-mediated DDIs detected, 215 (97%) had additional DDIs detected by the multidrug analysis software program that were not identified with use of the standard two-drug alert software program.[48] In sum, the multidrug software program identified a median increase of three (95% confidence interval, 2.5–3.5) potential CYP-mediated DDIs per patient and detected a total of 416 additional DDIs, compared with use of the standard two-drug software program.[48] By comparison, other researchers have observed poor performance of traditional drug alert software programs, in part by the failure of these programs to consistently detect and warn pharmacists and other health care professionals of well-documented, clinically relevant DDIs.[52,53,55,66] In a study designed to assess the performance of drug alert software programs used in 64 pharmacies in Arizona, overall, these programs failed to detect one in seven clinically significant DDIs.[55] These results are similar to an earlier conducted study, whereby researchers evaluated the performance of nine different drug alert software programs used in 516 pharmacies in Washington State. The software programs failed to detect clinically relevant DDIs one-third of the time.[66] Although there are few direct comparisons between the CYP-specific multidrug analysis software and traditional drug alert software programs, except for the aforesaid studies,[48,51] the consistently reported suboptimal performance of the latter addresses broader public safety concerns associated with the manner in which DDIs are detected and alerted within clinical decision support (CDS) systems and provides evidence that innovative strategies are needed to improve the performance of drug interaction tools.

In the previously mentioned study, using the multidrug analysis software program for a subsample of 52 geriatric patients, pharmacists targeted 12 (23%) of the patients for interventions, including medication discontinuation (three), medication substitution (three), dose adjustment (two), or close clinical monitoring (four).[48] Common reasons for pharmacist interventions to mitigate the risk of potential CYP-mediated DDIs were (1) when therapeutic failure or increased toxicity from one of the interacting CYP enzyme substrates was thought to underlie the condition that precipitated the patient's hospital admission (eg, uncontrolled neuropsychiatric symptoms in a patient with dementia), (2) when an equally effective alternative medication with a lower risk of potentially CYP-mediated DDIs was available at similar cost for a condition that required treatment, and (3) when one of the interacting medications had no clear indication for use.[48] Two examples of CYP-mediated DDIs that were judged by pharmacists to warrant intervention included diltiazem (CYP3A4 strong affinity substrate) plus simvastatin (CYP3A4 moderate affinity substrate), substitute simvastatin with rosuvastatin (metabolized by CYP2C9) to lessen myalgia caused by increased bioavailability and systemic concentrations of simvastatin as a result of competitive inhibition in a patient with muscle pain; and losartan (CYP3A4 prodrug) plus atorvastatin (CYP3A4 moderate affinity substrate) competitive inhibition, substitute losartan with valsartan (no hepatic metabolism) to increase therapeutic effectiveness in a patient with cardiovascular disease and uncontrolled lipids.[48]

Although only two-drug interactions are provided in these examples, other competing substrates for the same CYP enzymes were noted but judged by pharmacists to be of lesser clinical significance and, hence, not warrant intervention. In the absence of validation studies showing a consistent correlation between potential CYP-mediated DDIs and actual ADEs, MRM requires the pharmacist and prescriber to make a clinical judgment about the relevance of DDIs and need for medication changes, respectively. Notwithstanding, 15% of patients in this study had a change to their medication regimen as a result of the pharmacist interpretation of risk according to the interaction analysis matrix and their subsequent recommendations, and close clinical monitoring was recommended in an additional 8% of patients.[48] In an earlier study of the CYP-specific multidrug analysis software, researchers observed a higher (40%) intervention rate among specialized geriatric pharmacists.[51] This approximately one in three increased effort at DDI prevention, caused by use of the innovative multidrug software in busy pharmacies throughout the United States, represents an enhanced MTM strategy that could arguably be deemed clinically significant.

Future directions It is well known that DDIs are strongly associated with ADEs in geriatric populations.[67,68] By using multidrug analysis software programs, such as the one described in this section, pharmacists could determine the probability of a geriatric patient with polypharmacy experiencing a clinically important DDI that may potentially result in an ADE. Based on a single multidrug assessment rather than multiple sequential and potentially conflicting two-drug assessments, as is the traditional strategy of drug alert software programs, the expectation is that DDIs will be better predicted, not just recognized in a pairwise interaction, and that medication dose adjustments or alternatives will be made more prospectively, rather than reactively, to mitigate DDIs and the clinical sequelae of ADEs.[48]

Because pharmacists will likely continue to use validated tools to assess prescribing appropriateness for geriatric patients (eg, Beers Criteria), it is plausible that pairing such tools with multidrug analysis software programs could enhance medication decision-making and augment rates of safer medication management. For example, numerous reports indicate that some health care professionals and researchers criticize the application of the Beers Criteria to clinical practice for improving health outcomes,[69–72] whereas others are of the opinion that a medication is not clinically inappropriate for a specific geriatric patient merely because it is included in the Beers Criteria.[73] For example, according to the Beers Criteria, doxepin is a potentially inappropriate medication to use in all geriatric patients, regardless of medical condition, because of its significant anticholinergic and sedative properties and, hence, risk for causing or contributing to cognitive and physical impairment.[74] However, health care professionals may reasonably judge that doxepin is not clinically inappropriate to use for short-term management of insomnia in a geriatric patient in lieu of using a sedative hypnotic. Yet, if presented with DDI information from the multidrug analysis software program (eg, metoprolol and sertraline compete with doxepin for CYP2D6 and CYP2C19, respectively, thereby potentially increasing the systemic concentration of doxepin in this patient), one might surmise that most health care professionals would consider at least a dosage adjustment of doxepin (eg, reduced dosage), if not an alternative medication, for most geriatric patients with this DDI.

Many health care organizations and professionals endorse or use drug alert software programs to improve patient safety. Most interventions generated from these programs have been aimed at the prescriber.[75] Pharmacists may be better suited than prescribers to manage complex DDIs in geriatric patients. Research needs to evaluate how the two disciplines can work collaboratively to reduce the independent impact of DDIs during the already complex management of a geriatric patient's medications.[48] Also, research needs to determine the impact on health outcomes of incorporating innovative DDI support tools (ie, multidrug analysis software programs) into pharmacist-provided MTM, compared with usual care.

Pharmacogenomics

Background

It is well recognized that different patients respond in different ways to the same medication.[76] It is estimated that 25% of patients use at least one medication linked to altered response caused by genetic variants.[77–79] Furthermore, the results of an investigation of the top 200 medications most often prescribed in the United States suggest that the clinically well-established genetic variants of the CYP2C9, CYP2C19, and CYP2D6 enzymes may be relevant in almost 50% of the top 200 medications prescribed.[80] Commonly implicated medications and classes of medications include antidepressants, antipsychotics, β-blockers, clopidogrel, nonsteroidal anti-inflammatory drugs, and opioids.[78,80]

Although DDIs are a widely recognized major cause of ADEs, two other newly described important types of drug interactions also exist: the aforementioned DGIs and drug-drug-gene interactions (DDGIs). A DGI occurs when a patient's genetic CYP phenotype (eg, CYP2C19 intermediate metabolizer) affects that patient's ability to clear a drug or activate a pro-drug (eg, clopidogrel).[78] A DDGI occurs when a patient's genetic CYP phenotype and another drug in the patient's regimen (eg, a CYP2C19 strong affinity substrate or inhibitor) affect that patient's ability to clear a drug or activate a prodrug.[78] In a sample of 1143 patients (mean [± standard deviation] age, 60 [15] years; mean [± standard deviation] medications, 8.4 [5.7]) with known CYP2C9, CYP2C19, and CYP2D6 genotypes and phenotypes, researchers detected a total of 1053 potential major or substantial drug interactions among 501 patients. Each patient had, on average, 2.1 major or substantial drug interactions. DDIs accounted for 66.1% of the total interactions, whereas DGIs and DDGIs accounted for 14.7% and 19.2% of interactions, respectively.[78]

The promise of pharmacogenomics (PGx), the study of the relationship between genetic variants in a large collection of genes and variability in medication response, lies in its potential to predict which patients may respond to specific medications and to personalize medications for individual patients.[81,82] The concept of the medical utility of PGx to maximize the safety and effectiveness of medications aligns well with the goal of enhanced MTM to reduce ADEs and optimize therapeutic outcomes through improved medication use and personalized MTM services for geriatric patients. The concept also aligns nicely with the government's Precision Medicine Initiative, which is centered on tailoring a patient's care, including medication therapy, to their individual characteristics.

Evidence

PGx and personalized medicine are not new concepts. The idea of personalizing medications to a patient's unique genetic makeup has been extensively studied for the past 30 years.[83] However, for decades, PGx has been confined to the drug development and research realms. With more recent advancements in genetic technology and translational research, however, health care organizations, systems, and professionals in the United States are quickly beginning to embrace PGx, paving the way for this field of personalized medicine on a national scale.[82] Today, more than 150 medications include PGx information in their Food and Drug Administration–approved labeling.[84]

Various health care organizations and systems throughout the country are playing vital roles in the study and integration of PGx information into clinical practice.[85] These groups are collecting large amounts of data to understand genetic variants and responses to medications and translating the PGx information into real-world, clinical practice.[85] Although a detailed discussion of each of these health care organizations and systems is beyond the scope of this article, it is worth recognizing these groups for their cutting edge work in PGx. Health care organizations and systems paving the way for PGx include the following:

- 1200 Patients Project at the University of Chicago (https://cpt.uchicago.edu/page/1200-patients-project)[86]
- PG4KDS at St. Jude Children's Research Hospital (https://www.stjude.org/research/clinical-trials/pg4kds-pharmaceutical-science.html)[87]
- Pharmacogenomic Resource for Enhanced Decision in Care and Treatment at Vanderbilt University (http://www.mydruggenome.org/overview.php)[88]
- Personalized Medicine Program at the University of Florida (https://www.ctsi.ufl.edu/about/ctsi-programs/personalized-medicine/)[89–91]
- Program for Personalized and Genomic Medicine, including the Personalized Antiplatelet Pharmacogenetics Program, at the University of Maryland (http://medschool.umaryland.edu/genetics/)[92]
- Center for Individualized Medicine, including the Right Drug, Right Dose, Right Time–Using Genomic Data to Individualize Treatment Protocol, at the Mayo Clinic (http://mayoresearch.mayo.edu/center-for-individualized-medicine/pharmacogenomics-study.asp)[93]
- Indiana Institute of Personalized Medicine (https://iipm.medicinedept.iu.edu/)[94]

Improved scientific understanding of the interplay between genetics and medication response provides pharmacists, as medication management experts, with information to predict which geriatric patients may respond safely and effectively to a particular medication. Building from the evolving collaborative role of pharmacists through MTM services, the application for pharmacists to use PGx information in clinical practice to improve patient care is emerging.[95] A growing body of research is providing evidence for pharmacist-provided PGx clinical services, especially as part of MTM services.[77,90,96–102] Notwithstanding this progress, research in this area has been largely comprised of feasibility studies; albeit, as with any new service, integration requires careful planning and evaluating.

Future directions
Integrating PGx information into the clinical decision-making process has the potential to improve medication adherence, effectiveness, and safety, and therapeutic outcomes for geriatric patients.[90] The ability to integrate PGx information into clinical practice is a reasonable extension of existing pharmacy services,[77] as evidenced by the growing body of research of pharmacist-provided PGx clinical services. Integrating PGx into pharmacy practice as part of MTM services may prove to be more effective than traditional MTM alone. However, the effectiveness of the integration has not yet been determined.[103]

INTEGRATING ENHANCED MEDICATION RISK MITIGATION STRATEGIES INTO CLINICAL PRACTICE

Although MTM services address many of the factors affecting medication response in geriatric patients,[104,105] such as the number and types of medications prescribed, traditionally, these services use a one-size-fits-all strategy, which is largely because of the regulatory inflexibility and stringent criteria imposed by CMS for MTM programs. With the recently conceptualized Enhanced MTM Model, pharmacists have an opportunity to transform the one-size-fits-all strategy to medication management into a geriatric patient-specific strategy. Nevertheless, mitigating medication risk for geriatric patients is complex, and successful strategies often are labor intensive and multilayered. As pharmacists, and other health care professionals, embark on developing patient-specific and enhanced MTM strategies, it is important to understand the challenges to integrating these strategies that may lay ahead.

FOCUS ON PHARMACOGENOMICS

This section focuses on integrating PGx into clinical practice as a potential innovative strategy for the Enhanced MTM Model. Although there has been substantial hype over the promise of PGx in personalized medicine and to mitigate medication risk, PGx has only recently begun to be integrated into actual clinical practice. Overall, the speed of the discovery of genetic variants far outpaces the understanding of corresponding clinical significance.[84] Notwithstanding the scientific pace, the lag in integrating PGx into clinical practice may be caused, in part, by an appreciable number of barriers. Understanding these barriers and devising enabling strategies to overcome them not only requires careful consideration of effects on health care systems, prescribing practices, and patient behaviors, but is necessary for PGx to achieve its true potential and imperative for developing successful and sustainable MTM models that include PGx as part of their service offerings.

Barriers to Integration

We compiled a list of barriers to integrating PGx into clinical practice from various resources, including the primary literature (**Box 1**). Overall, barriers include health care system-, patient-, and health care professional–related barriers.

Health care system–related barriers

One health care system–related barrier involves the uniqueness of PGx data compared with other commonly interpreted data in the electronic health record (EHR).[85] This includes the massive size of PGx data, which may require the development of an interface to integrate an external data warehouse to the EHR; complicated algorithms and processes required to translate random sequence numbers and single nucleotide polymorphisms into genotypes and actionable phenotypes; the ever-changing interpretation of PGx data; and the need to store and make PGx data accessible throughout patients' lives.[85] Determining how to code and interpret PGx data for integration in the EHR requires multidisciplinary collaboration that includes pharmacists.[85]

Patient-related barriers

Although patients seem genuinely interested in PGx testing, they have concerns. A US survey of public attitudes toward PGx testing confirmed that most patients are not likely to consent to having a PGx test if they perceive a risk that their DNA sample or test result could be shared without their permission.[108] Other public surveys and focus groups have revealed that patients are concerned about ancillary information (eg, unexpected disease risk) unrelated to the purpose for which the test was ordered.[119,120] Given these concerns, health care professionals should clearly discuss with patients the purpose of PGx testing, the benefits and risks of testing, and policies to protect confidentiality and privacy.

Health care professional–related barriers

A barrier at the health care professional–level that is addressable is gaps in knowledge (about the science) and competency (about the clinical application) of PGx. Studies and surveys of licensed health care professionals have revealed that most lack sufficient knowledge about the topic of PGx and are not competent to integrate it into

Box 1
Barriers and enablers for integrating pharmacogenomics into clinical practice

Barriers

Health Care System–Related Barriers[77,85,95,103,106,107]
- Uniqueness of PGx data compared with other commonly interpreted data in the EHR
- Lack of system capacity to store PGx data
- Lack of sophisticated CDS systems to translate PGx data into information for medical decision-making
- No standardized terminology specifically designated for documenting PGx information
- Poor interoperability/lack of capability to transfer PGx data between systems and to follow the patient across health care systems
- Incorporating PGx information into health care professionals' workflow and busy schedules
- Little cost-benefit or cost-effectiveness on PGx testing and value
- Partnering with a PGx laboratory/actually ordering a PGx test
- Insurance coverage restrictions/lack of reimbursement from third-party payers for PGx testing and for MTM services associated with the test
- Delay/slow turnaround time of receiving PGx test results for making optimal decisions

Patient-Related Barriers[95,108]
- Insufficient understanding of PGx and appreciation of the benefits of PGx
- Concerns about genetic testing and what should be tested
- Concerns about patient privacy and confidentiality
- Concerns about the personal implications of learning about ancillary information (eg, unexpected disease risk)
- Concerns about whether PGx test results will be shared with the patient and/or follow the patient throughout the health care system

Health Care Professional–Related Barriers[77,95,98,103,107,109–117]
- Knowledge and competency gaps for health care professionals
- Need for continuing education as PGx grows
- Perception of PGx as a low priority in clinical practice
- Concerns about the lack of evidence of clinical utility of PGx
- Time (often substantial) required to analyze, interpret, communicate, and make clinical decisions based on the results of PGx testing
- Disagreement/misalignment on how to appropriately assign clinical responsibility for actionable PGx results
- Limited access to patient's EHR, or at least care-oriented data, such as laboratory data and problem lists (eg, pharmacists, especially in community practice)
- Unable to order PGx testing (eg, pharmacists, because of nonrecognized provider status)

Enablers

Health Care System–Related Enablers[77,85,93,95,106,118,119]
- Development of a unique, easily accessible location within an EHR user interface or third-party application to store PGx data
- CDS integrated into the EHR
- Developing and using standardized terminology to allow PGx information to be sent to other health care systems using certified EHR software via HIE
- Publicly accessible PGx databases (eg, PharmGKB)
- Clinical practice guidelines for medication selection and dose adjustment, when PGx information is available (eg, CPIC, DPWG)
- Preemptive PGx testing
- Availability of point-of-care PGx tests

Patient-Related Enablers[77,86,97,98,108]
- Patient interest in PGx information is robust

Health Care Professional–Related Enablers[77,95]
- Use of pharmacists to interpret and apply PGx information
- Prescriber adoption of PGx information, when accessible and interpretable, is high

- Advanced practice designation for nonproviders (eg, pharmacists), such as CPP, with ordering or prescribing privileges under a CPA or SOP

Abbreviations: CPA, collaborative practice agreement; CPIC, Clinical Pharmacogenetics Implementation Consortium; CPP, clinical pharmacist practitioner; DPWG, Dutch Pharmacogenetic Working Group; EHR, electronic health record; HIE, health information exchange; PharmGKB, pharmacogenomics knowledgebase; SOP, scope of practice.
Data from Refs.[77,85,86,93,95,97,98,103,106–118]

clinical practice.[110,121] These knowledge and competency gaps have not escaped the public's attention. For example, a national poll of 1000 US adults revealed that greater than 80% lacked confidence in their physician's ability to understand and use genomic information in clinical practice.[122] Colleges and universities could play a pivotal role in educating health care professionals on the latest developments and optimal applications in PGx.[109] Yet, multiple studies assessing the extent and depth of PGx instruction in the professional curricula of colleges and universities in the United States have exposed that a great deal of work needs to be done to expand PGx education.[109,116,123,124] For example, a survey of PGx instruction in colleges and universities of pharmacy revealed that although 78% of the sample provides some instruction in PGx, which demonstrates an awareness of the importance of this field to pharmacy, the depth of education on the topic is suboptimal.[109] According to the survey, the sample providing PGx instruction is only addressing about 30% to 50% of the American Association of Colleges of Pharmacy Academic Affairs Committee's recommendations on pharmacist knowledge and competency for this field.[108] Collectively, these knowledge and competency gaps have been cited as substantial barriers to the integration of PGx into clinical practice.[111,112]

Enablers for Integration

Barriers exist, but there are unprecedented opportunities for health care professionals, researchers, and universities to collaborate to lead the integration of PGx into the US health care system. Enablers for integrating PGx into clinical practice also are listed in **Box 1**, alongside the barriers. Similarly, enablers include health care system–, patient–, and health care professional–related enablers.

Health care system–related enablers

From a health care system perspective, there are several enablers. One enabler is the diverse databases and guidelines that are publicly accessible to health care professionals, universities, and researchers for the rapidly growing field of PGx. Some of the pharmacy-specific resources are listed next. These databases and guidelines are necessary to make the integration of PGx information into clinical practice possible.[85]

- Pharmacogenomics Knowledgebase (https://www.pharmgkb.org/)
- Clinical Pharmacogenetics Implementation Consortium (https://cpicpgx.org/)
- Dutch Pharmacogenetic Working Group (https://www.pharmgkb.org/page/dpwg)
- Electronic Medical Records and Genomics Network (https://www.genome.gov/27540473/electronic-medical-records-and-genomics-emerge-network/)
- Implementing Genomics in Practice Consortium (https://www.genome.gov/27554264/implementing-genomics-in-practice-ignite/)

Patient-related enablers

Although information on patient-related enablers is scarce in comparison with health care system– and professional-related enablers, available research consistently demonstrates that patients are generally interested and willing to participate in PGx testing, particularly pharmacy- or pharmacist-initiated testing.[77,97,98] In a survey of US public attitudes toward PGx testing, approximately 70% to 90% of respondents expressed interest in PGx testing.[108] In the pharmacy practice setting, several studies demonstrated that about 50% to 80% of patients who qualified for PGx testing gave informed consent to be tested.[77,97,98] Factors that may affect patients' interest and willingness to participate in PGx testing include trust in health care professionals, level of education, location in relation to academic community, perceived invasiveness of the test, and out-of-pocket cost.[77,98]

Health care professional–related enablers

Pharmacists currently are providing MTM services, in diverse health care settings, to help patients avoid ADEs and achieve positive therapeutic outcomes. A PGx service is an enhancement to MTM services, which would certainly enable the integration of PGx into clinical practice.[77,95,96] Recognizing the valuable roles that PGx information and pharmacists can play in mitigating medication risk and optimizing medication effectiveness, pharmacy organizations, such as the American Pharmacists Association and American Society of Health-System Pharmacists, have begun to define the pharmacist's role in integrating PGx into clinical practice through MTM.[95,125] Confirmatory information about the pharmacist's role in integrating PGx into clinical practice is garnered from researchers that have begun to study such integration. The role of pharmacists in integrating PGx into clinical practice may include the following[77,90,95,125,126]:

- Perform sample collection, particularly of buccal or saliva samples, to be used for PGx testing
- Work collaboratively with laboratory professionals to interpret PGx data to determine actionable phenotypes for medication selection and dosing and, if needed, suggest alternative medications to prescribers
- Collaborate with health care professionals to define processes and workflows to bring the promise of PGx to patients
- Incorporate PGx information into the EHR to assist with collaboration between health care professionals and medication decision-making
- Encourage and participate in the development and implementation of health information technology solutions, including CDS systems, that use PGx information to optimize and personalize medications for patients
- Educate health care professionals, patients, and members of the public about PGx
- Support and participate in consortia, networks, and research that guide and accelerate the application of PGx to clinical practice
- Develop processes to document improved patient outcomes and economic benefits resulting from applied PGx
- Contribute to the body of knowledge and evidence in PGx by publishing articles on the topic in the biomedical literature
- Work with advocacy and collaborative groups (eg, Pharmacy e-Health Information Technology Collaborative) to pursue EHR standards that support the provision and payment of pharmacist-provided PGx services

As a compliment to patients' interest and willingness to participate in PGx testing, research also suggests that prescribers are accepting of PGx-based recommendations, particularly from pharmacists.[77] Moreover, research suggests that prescribers are more accepting of pharmacist-provided, PGx-based recommendations than traditional MTM-based recommendations. In one PGx service integration study in the outpatient setting, prescribers accepted nearly 90% of pharmacists' recommendations for continuation or modification of medication therapy.[77] However, traditional MTM intervention studies in the outpatient setting have found prescriber acceptance rates between 40% and 60%.[127–130]

POWER OF INTEGRATION

To demonstrate the power of integrating PGx with multidrug analysis, the following case study illustrates complex DDI, DGI, and DDGI that may occur in a geriatric patient.

Patient Case Scenario

A 72-year-old male patient with a past medical history of cardiovascular disease and myocardial infarction is presently managed with the following medications: metoprolol, 100 mg orally twice daily; amitriptyline, 100 mg orally at bedtime; clopidogrel, 150 mg orally twice daily; pantoprazole, 40 mg orally daily; and atorvastatin, 40 mg orally at bedtime. His PGx test results reveal the following: CYP2C19*17|*17, CYP2D6*1|*1, and CYP3A4*1|*1.

The pharmacist's interpretation of his PGx test results is that the patient is an ultra-rapid metabolizer of CYP2C19, a normal metabolizer of CYP2D6, and an extensive metabolizer of CYP3A4. Surprisingly, the patient is on a high dose of clopidogrel, a prodrug, which should be more extensively converted to its active metabolite given that the patient is an ultrarapid metabolizer of CYP2C19.

Side effects are observed from amitriptyline (eg, intolerable constipation and dry eyes, cognitive decline), which is discontinued, and paroxetine, 20 mg orally daily, is introduced into the patient's medication regimen. Additionally, atorvastatin is replaced with pravastatin, 40 mg orally at bedtime because the patient complains of muscle pain.

Patient Case Explanation

First, refer to **Fig. 1** (*part A*) for an explanation of amitriptyline. Metoprolol and amitriptyline are both substrates of the CYP2D6 enzyme, as indicated by the color coding in the cell. However, metoprolol has much higher affinity than amitriptyline for this CYP enzyme, as indicated by the darker color in the metoprolol cell. Amitriptyline clearance could be decreased by 35%, as indicated by the extent of drug metabolism by CYP2D6 for amitriptyline. Therefore, although the patient is a normal metabolizer of CYP2D6 for metoprolol, because of phenoconversion, he became a poor metabolizer for amitriptyline. As a result, metoprolol inhibited the metabolism (hydroxylation) of amitriptyline to its inactive metabolite (10-hydroxy amitriptyline).

Amitriptyline is converted to nortriptyline by the CYP2C19 enzyme. Because the patient is an ultrarapid metabolizer of CYP2C19, one would have expected higher systemic concentrations of nortriptyline. However, because pantoprazole also is a substrate of the CYP2C19 enzyme, competitive inhibition is observed between these two substrates, leading to decreased clearances and increased plasma levels of both drugs (especially for pantoprazole, because 90% of its clearances is through CYP2C19). As a result, pantoprazole-mediated inhibition of CYP2C19 decreased the demethylation of amitriptyline and formation of its active metabolite (nortriptyline).

During the final phase of its metabolic pathway, the active metabolite of amitriptyline (nortriptyline) is metabolized by the CYP3A4 enzyme to undergo renal excretion. Atorvastatin also is a substrate of the CYP3A4 enzyme, but it has much higher affinity than

Medication	ACB	SDB	F%	Ae%	CYP2C19 *17|*17	CYP2D6 *1|*1	CYP3A4 *1|*1
Part A – Initial Medication Regimen							
Pantoprazole	0	1	77	0	90		
Metoprolol	1	1	50	5		80	
Clopidogrel	0	0	1	0	10ᵃ		5ᵃ
Atorvastatin	0	0	13	0.1			80
Amitriptyline	3	3	48	5	30	35	10
Part B – Revised Medication Regimen							
Pantoprazole	0	1	77	0	90		
Metoprolol	1	1	50	5		80	
Clopidogrel	0	0	1	0	10ᵃ		5ᵃ
Pravastatin	0	1	17	23			10
Paroxetine	3	2	50	2		70	

□ = CYP weak affinity substrate, ▢ = CYP moderate affinity substrate, ▣ = CYP strong affinity substrate, ■ = CYP inhibitor. The number in the cells for CYP450 isoenzymes indicates the extent this isoenzyme contributes to the overall clearance of the drug.

Fig. 1. Patient case scenario using the multidrug analysis software. ACB, anticholinergic cognitive burden; Ae, amount excreted in urine (%); F, absolute bioavailability (%); SDB, sedative burden. ᵃ Prodrug (ie, clopidogrel). (© 2016 Tabula Rasa HealthCare, Inc. All Rights Reserved.)

amitriptyline for this CYP enzyme, as indicated by the darker color in the atorvastatin cell. Therefore, although the patient is a normal metabolizer of CYP3A4 for atorvastatin, because of phenoconversion, he became a poor metabolizer for nortriptyline. As a result, atorvastatin inhibited the renal excretion of nortriptyline. Unrelated to its metabolism, amitriptyline has strong anticholinergic properties; as denoted by a score of 3 (out of 3) in **Fig. 1**. The net result of this multidrug-gene interaction is that the systemic concentrations of amitriptyline were much higher than expected, which likely caused or contributed to the anticholinergic side effects the patient experienced.

Next, refer to **Fig. 1** (*part A*) for an explanation of clopidogrel. Clopidogrel is sequentially metabolized to its active metabolite by several CYP enzymes, most notably CYP2C19 but also including CYP3A4. Because the patient is an ultrarapid metabolizer of clopidogrel by the CYP2C19 enzyme, one would have expected an increase in the formation of its active metabolite. However, there was competitive inhibition at both the CYP2C19 enzyme (ie, pantoprazole and amitriptyline) and CYP3A4 enzyme (ie, atorvastatin), resulting in phenoconversion of these enzymes (eg, CYP2C19 ultrarapid to intermediate or poor metabolizer; CYP3A4 normal to poor metabolizer). As a result, there was a net decrease in the formation of the clopidogrel active metabolite, which could have resulted in therapeutic failure. This may explain why the patient is on an exceptionally high dose of clopidogrel.

Finally, refer to **Fig. 1** (*part B*) for an explanation of the recent changes to the patient's medications. When amitriptyline and atorvastatin were switched to different medications, the aforementioned conversion of clopidogrel to its active metabolite would have increased. As a result, if the dose of clopidogrel is not subsequently decreased, the patient will be at increased risk for bleeding. When paroxetine was added, because it is both a strong substrate for and inhibitor (via formation of a metabolite complex) of the CYP2D6 enzyme, phenoconversion would have taken place and the patient would become a poor metabolizer for metoprolol. As a result, the patient is at increased risk for metoprolol-related side effects (eg, bradycardia, hypotension) at his current dose.

Although some of the overall medication risks have been mitigated, such as anticholinergic side effects from amitriptyline, paroxetine has strong anticholinergic properties as well, as denoted by a score of 3 (out of 3) in **Fig. 1**. Thus, the patient is still at high risk for experiencing anticholinergic side effects, which may warrant further intervention.

SUMMARY

The current high prevalence of MRPs and ADEs in geriatric populations is unacceptable, and represents a public health problem likely to grow in tandem with aging populations. Traditional MRM strategies have proven to be effective at mitigating medication risk, but these strategies have not consistently translated into positive health outcomes for geriatric populations. Enhanced MRM strategies are needed and these strategies need to be tested to assess their impact on the incidence of ADEs and other clinical, humanistic, and economic outcomes in this vulnerable population. A formidable challenge for health care systems and professionals is successfully integrating enhanced MRM strategies, such as PGx information, into clinical practice. As one of the most trusted and accessible health care professionals in the United States and the medication experts on health care teams, pharmacists have a clear role to play in developing, integrating, and assessing enhanced MRM strategies to reduce ADEs and improve therapeutic outcomes for geriatric patients.

ACKNOWLEDGMENTS

The authors and editors thank Dr Roland Valdes and Dr Erik Korte for their time and review of this article.

REFERENCES

1. Viswanathan M, Kahwati LC, Golin CE, et al. Medication therapy management interventions in outpatient settings. Comparative effectiveness review No. 138. (Prepared by the RTI International–University of North Carolina at Chapel Hill evidence-based practice center under contract No. 290-2012-00008-I.) AHRQ Publication No. 14(15)-EHC037-EF. Rockville (MD): Agency for Healthcare Research and Quality; 2014. Available at: www.effectivehealthcare.ahrq.gov/reports/final.cfm. Accessed August 10, 2015.
2. Kohn LT, Corrigan JM, Donaldson MS, editors. To err is human: building a safer health system. Washington, DC: National Academy Press; 2000.
3. McGlynn EA, Asch SM, Adams J, et al. The quality of health care delivered to adults in the United States. N Engl J Med 2003;348(26):2635–45.
4. Cooper JA, Cadogan CA, Patterson SM, et al. Interventions to improve the appropriate use of polypharmacy in older people: a Cochrane systematic review. BMJ Open 2015;5(12):e009235.
5. Marcum ZA, Amuan ME, Hanlon JT, et al. Prevalence of unplanned hospitalizations caused by adverse drug reactions in older veterans. J Am Geriatr Soc 2012;60(1):34–41.
6. Cahir C, Fahey T, Teeling M, et al. Potentially inappropriate prescribing and cost outcomes for older people: a national population study. Br J Clin Pharmacol 2010;69(5):543–52.

7. Bradley MC, Fahey T, Cahir C, et al. Potentially inappropriate prescribing and cost outcomes for older people: a cross-sectional study using the Northern Ireland Enhanced Prescribing Database. Eur J Clin Pharmacol 2012;68(10): 1425–33.

8. Hajjar ER, Hanlon JT, Artz MB, et al. Adverse drug reaction risk factors in older outpatients. Am J Geriatr Pharmacother 2003;1(2):82–9.

9. Maher RL, Hanlon J, Hajjar ER. Clinical consequences of polypharmacy in elderly. Expert Opin Drug Saf 2014;13(1):57–65.

10. Budnitz DS, Shehab N, Kegler SR, et al. Medication use leading to emergency department visits for adverse drug events in older adults. Ann Intern Med 2007; 147(11):755–65.

11. Budnitz DS, Lovegrove MC, Shehab N, et al. Emergency hospitalizations for adverse drug events in older Americans. N Engl J Med 2011;365(21):2002–12.

12. Kongkaew C, Noyce PR, Ashcroft DM. Hospital admissions associated with adverse drug reactions: a systematic review of prospective observational studies. Ann Pharmacother 2008;42(7):1017–25.

13. Fulton MM, Allen ER. Polypharmacy in the elderly: a literature review. J Am Acad Nurse Pract 2005;17(4):123–32.

14. Hamilton HJ, Gallagher PF, O'Mahony D. Inappropriate prescribing and adverse drug events in older people. BMC Geriatr 2009;9:5.

15. Beijer HJ, de Blaey CJ. Hospitalisations caused by adverse drug reactions (ADR): a meta-analysis of observational studies. Pharm World Sci 2002;24(2): 46–54.

16. Chan M, Nicklason F, Vial JH. Adverse drug events as a cause of hospital admission in the elderly. Intern Med J 2001;31(4):199–205.

17. Classen DC, Pestotnik SL, Evans RS, et al. Adverse drug events in hospitalized patients. Excess length of stay, extra costs, and attributable mortality. JAMA 1997;277(4):301–6.

18. Tangiisuran B, Wright J, Van der Cammen T, et al. Adverse drug reactions in elderly: challenges in identification and improving preventative strategies. Age Ageing 2009;38(4):358–9.

19. Pretorius RW, Gataric G, Swedlund SK, et al. Reducing the risk of adverse drug events in older adults. Am Fam Physician 2013;87(5):331–6.

20. Bates DW, Leape LL, Petrycki S. Incidence and preventability of adverse drug events in hospitalized adults. J Gen Intern Med 1993;8(6):289–94.

21. Moore JM, Shartle D, Faudskar L, et al. Impact of a patient-centered pharmacy program and intervention in a high-risk group. J Manag Care Pharm 2013;19(3): 228–36.

22. Avalere health. Exploring pharmacists' role in a changing healthcare environment. Washington, DC: Avalere Health, LLC; 2014. Available at: http://www.nacds.org/pdfs/comm/2014/pharmacist-role.pdf. Accessed September 18, 2015.

23. Midwest Pharmacy Research Consortium. 2014 national pharmacist workforce survey. Minneapolis (MN): University of Minnesota; 2015. Available at: http://www.aacp.org/resources/research/pharmacyworkforcecenter/Documents/FinalReportOfTheNationalPharmacistWorkforceStudy2014.pdf. Accessed April 7, 2016.

24. Bluml BM. Definition of medication therapy management: development of professionwide consensus. J Am Pharm Assoc (2003) 2005;45(5):566–72.

25. American Pharmacists Association and National Association of Chain Drug Stores Foundation. Medication therapy management in pharmacy practice: core elements of an MTM service model version 2.0. Washington, DC: American

Pharmacists Association; 2008. Available at: http://www.pharmacist.com/sites/default/files/files/core_elements_of_an_mtm_practice.pdf. Accessed September 18, 2015.

26. Ryan R, Santesso N, Lowe D, et al. Interventions to improve safe and effective medicines use by consumers: an overview of systematic reviews. Cochrane Database Syst Rev 2014;(4):CD007768.

27. Alldred DP, Raynor DK, Hughes C, et al. Interventions to optimise prescribing for older people in care homes. Cochrane Database Syst Rev 2013;(2):CD009095.

28. Perlroth D, Marrufo G, Montesinos A, et al. Medication therapy management in chronically Ill populations. (Prepared by Acumen, LLC under contract No. HHSM-500-2011-00012I/TOT0.). Baltimore (MD): Centers for Medicare & Medicaid Services (CMS), Center for Medicare & Medicaid Innovation; 2013. Available at: https://innovation.cms.gov/files/reports/mtm_final_report.pdf. Accessed September 18, 2015.

29. Academy of Managed Care Pharmacy, Shoemaker SJ, Pozniak A, et al. Effect of 6 managed care pharmacy tools: a review of the literature. J Manag Care Pharm 2010;16(6 Suppl):S3–20.

30. Holland R, Desborough J, Goodyer L, et al. Does pharmacist-led medication review help to reduce hospital admissions and deaths in older people? A systematic review and meta-analysis. Br J Clin Pharmacol 2008;65(3):303–16.

31. O'Dell KM, Kucukarslan SN. Impact of the clinical pharmacist on readmission in patients with acute coronary syndrome. Ann Pharmacother 2005;39(9):1423–7.

32. Zillich AJ, Jaynes HA, Snyder ME, et al. Evaluation of specialized medication packaging combined with medication therapy management: adherence, outcomes, and costs among Medicaid patients. Med Care 2012;50(6):485–93.

33. Wittayanukorn S, Westrick SC, Hansen RA, et al. Evaluation of medication therapy management services for patients with cardiovascular disease in a self-insured employer health plan. J Manag Care Pharm 2013;19(5):385–95.

34. Gattis WA, Hasselblad V, Whellan DJ, et al. Reduction in heart failure events by the addition of a clinical pharmacist to the heart failure management team: results of the Pharmacist in Heart Failure Assessment Recommendation and Monitoring (PHARM) Study. Arch Intern Med 1999;159(16):1939–45.

35. Lee AJ, Boro MS, Knapp KK, et al. Clinical and economic outcomes of pharmacist recommendations in a Veterans Affairs medical center. Am J Health Syst Pharm 2002;59(21):2070–7.

36. Isetts BJ, Schondelmeyer SW, Artz MB, et al. Clinical and economic outcomes of medication therapy management services: the Minnesota experience. J Am Pharm Assoc (2003) 2008;48(2):203–11.

37. Fox D, Ried LD, Klein GE, et al. A medication therapy management program's impact on low-density lipoprotein cholesterol goal attainment in Medicare Part D patients with diabetes. J Am Pharm Assoc (2003) 2009;49(2):192–9.

38. Pindolia VK, Stebelsky L, Romain TM, et al. Mitigation of medication mishaps via medication therapy management. Ann Pharmacother 2009;43(4):611–20.

39. Welch EK, Delate T, Chester EA, et al. Assessment of the impact of medication therapy management delivered to home-based Medicare beneficiaries. Ann Pharmacother 2009;43(4):603–10.

40. Robinson JD, Segal R, Lopez LM, et al. Impact of a pharmaceutical care intervention on blood pressure control in a chain pharmacy practice. Ann Pharmacother 2010;44(1):88–96.

41. Pape GA, Hunt JS, Butler KL, et al. Team-based care approach to cholesterol management in diabetes mellitus: two-year cluster randomized controlled trial. Arch Intern Med 2011;171(16):1480–6.

42. Okamoto MP, Nakahiro RK. Pharmacoeconomic evaluation of a pharmacist-managed hypertension clinic. Pharmacotherapy 2001;21(11):1337–44.

43. Isetts BJ, Schondelmeyer SW, Heaton AH, et al. Effects of collaborative drug therapy management on patients' perceptions of care and health-related quality of life. Res Social Adm Pharm 2006;2(1):129–42.

44. Schumock GT, Butler MG, Meek PD, et al. Evidence of the economic benefit of clinical pharmacy services: 1996-2000. Pharmacotherapy 2003;23(1):113–32.

45. Trygstad TK, Christensen DB, Wegner SE, et al. Analysis of the North Carolina long-term care polypharmacy initiative: a multiple-cohort approach using propensity-score matching for both evaluation and targeting. Clin Ther 2009; 31(9):2018–37.

46. Viswanathan M, Kahwati LC, Golin CE, et al. Medication therapy management interventions in outpatient settings: a systematic review and meta-analysis. JAMA Intern Med 2015;175(1):76–87.

47. Centers for Medicare & Medicaid Services. CMS announces Part D Enhanced Medication Therapy Management Model. 2015. Available at: https://www.cms. gov/Newsroom/MediaReleaseDatabase/Press-releases/2015-Press-releases-items/2015-09-28.html. Accessed September 29, 2015.

48. Doan J, Zakrzewski-Jakubiak H, Roy J, et al. Prevalence and risk of potential cytochrome P450-mediated drug-drug interactions in older hospitalized patients with polypharmacy. Ann Pharmacother 2013;47(3):324–32.

49. Tannenbaum C, Sheehan NL. Understanding and preventing drug-drug and drug-gene interactions. Expert Rev Clin Pharmacol 2014;7(4):533–44.

50. Davies SJ, Eayrs S, Pratt P, et al. Potential for drug interactions involving cytochromes P450 2D6 and 3A4 on general adult psychiatric and functional elderly psychiatric wards. Br J Clin Pharmacol 2004;57(4):464–72.

51. Zakrzewski-Jakubiak H, Doan J, Lamoureux P, et al. Detection and prevention of drug-drug interactions in the hospitalized elderly: utility of new cytochrome p450-based software. Am J Geriatr Pharmacother 2011;9(6):461–70.

52. Sweidan M, Reeve JF, Brien JA, et al. Quality of drug interaction alerts in prescribing and dispensing software. Med J Aust 2009;190(5):251–4.

53. Abarca J, Colon LR, Wang VS, et al. Evaluation of the performance of drug-drug interaction screening software in community and hospital pharmacies. J Manag Care Pharm 2006;12(5):383–9.

54. Tilson H, Hines LE, McEvoy G, et al. Recommendations for selecting drug-drug interactions for clinical decision support. Am J Health Syst Pharm 2016;73(8): 576–85.

55. Saverno KR, Hines LE, Warholak TL, et al. Ability of pharmacy clinical decision-support software to alert users about clinically important drug-drug interactions. J Am Med Inform Assoc 2011;18(1):32–7.

56. Lapane KL, Waring ME, Schneider KL, et al. A mixed method study of the merits of e-prescribing drug alerts in primary care. J Gen Intern Med 2008;23(4): 442–6.

57. Shah NR, Seger AC, Seger DL, et al. Improving acceptance of computerized prescribing alerts in ambulatory care. J Am Med Inform Assoc 2006;13(1):5–11.

58. Weingart SN, Simchowitz B, Shiman L, et al. Clinicians' assessments of electronic medication safety alerts in ambulatory care. Arch Intern Med 2009; 169(17):1627–32.

59. van der Sijs H, Aarts J, Vulto A, et al. Overriding of drug safety alerts in computerized physician order entry. J Am Med Inform Assoc 2006;13(2):138–47.

60. Isaac T, Weissman JS, Davis RB, et al. Overrides of medication alerts in ambulatory care. Arch Intern Med 2009;169(3):305–11.

61. Bryant AD, Fletcher GS, Payne TH. Drug interaction alert override rates in the Meaningful Use era: no evidence of progress. Appl Clin Inform 2014;5(3): 802–13.

62. Roe S, Long R, King K. Pharmacies miss half of dangerous drug combinations. Chicago Tribune. 2016. Available at: http://www.chicagotribune.com/news/watchdog/druginteractions/ct-drug-interactions-pharmacy-met-20161214-story.html. Accessed December 19, 2016.

63. Cavuto NJ, Woosley RL, Sale M. Pharmacies and prevention of potentially fatal drug interactions. JAMA 1996;275(14):1086–7.

64. Dimitrow MS, Airaksinen MS, Kivela SL, et al. Comparison of prescribing criteria to evaluate the appropriateness of drug treatment in individuals aged 65 and older: a systematic review. J Am Geriatr Soc 2011;59(8):1521–30.

65. Bulloch MN, Olin JL. Instruments for evaluating medication use and prescribing in older adults. J Am Pharm Assoc (2003) 2014;54(5):530–7.

66. Hazlet TK, Lee TA, Hansten PD, et al. Performance of community pharmacy drug interaction software. J Am Pharm Assoc (Wash) 2001;41(2):200–4.

67. Mallet L, Spinewine A, Huang A. The challenge of managing drug interactions in elderly people. Lancet 2007;370(9582):185–91.

68. Hines LE, Murphy JE. Potentially harmful drug-drug interactions in the elderly: a review. Am J Geriatr Pharmacother 2011;9(6):364–77.

69. Page RL 2nd, Ruscin JM. The risk of adverse drug events and hospital-related morbidity and mortality among older adults with potentially inappropriate medication use. Am J Geriatr Pharmacother 2006;4(4):297–305.

70. Laroche ML, Charmes JP, Nouaille Y, et al. Is inappropriate medication use a major cause of adverse drug reactions in the elderly? Br J Clin Pharmacol 2007;63(2):177–86.

71. Hanlon JT, Fillenbaum GG, Kuchibhatla M, et al. Impact of inappropriate drug use on mortality and functional status in representative community dwelling elders. Med Care 2002;40(2):166–76.

72. Hamilton H, Gallagher P, Ryan C, et al. Potentially inappropriate medications defined by STOPP criteria and the risk of adverse drug events in older hospitalized patients. Arch Intern Med 2011;171(11):1013–9.

73. Bain KT, Weschules DJ. Medication inappropriateness for older adults receiving hospice care: a pilot survey. Consult Pharm 2007;22(11):926–34.

74. American Geriatrics Society 2015 Beers Criteria Update Expert Panel. American geriatrics Society 2015 updated Beers criteria for potentially inappropriate medication use in older adults. J Am Geriatr Soc 2015;63(11):2227–46.

75. McKibbon KA, Lokker C, Handler SM, et al. The effectiveness of integrated health information technologies across the phases of medication management: a systematic review of randomized controlled trials. J Am Med Inform Assoc 2012;19(1):22–30.

76. Evans WE, McLeod HL. Pharmacogenomics: drug disposition, drug targets, and side effects. N Engl J Med 2003;348(6):538–49.

77. Ferreri SP, Greco AJ, Michaels NM, et al. Implementation of a pharmacogenomics service in a community pharmacy. J Am Pharm Assoc (2003) 2014;54(2): 172–80.

78. Verbeurgt P, Mamiya T, Oesterheld J. How common are drug and gene interactions? Prevalence in a sample of 1143 patients with CYP2C9, CYP2C19 and CYP2D6 genotyping. Pharmacogenomics 2014;15(5):655–65.
79. Grice GR, Seaton TL, Woodland AM, et al. Defining the opportunity for pharmacogenetic intervention in primary care. Pharmacogenomics 2006;7(1):61–5.
80. Zanger UM, Turpeinen M, Klein K, et al. Functional pharmacogenetics/genomics of human cytochromes P450 involved in drug biotransformation. Anal Bioanal Chem 2008;392(6):1093–108.
81. Cardelli M, Marchegiani F, Corsonello A, et al. A review of pharmacogenetics of adverse drug reactions in elderly people. Drug Saf 2012;35(Suppl 1):3–20.
82. Beier MT, Panchapagesan M, Carman LE. Pharmacogenetics: has the time come for pharmacists to embrace and implement the science? Consult Pharm 2013;28(11):696–711.
83. Crettol S, de Leon J, Hiemke C, et al. Pharmacogenomics in psychiatry: from therapeutic drug monitoring to genomic medicine. Clin Pharmacol Ther 2014; 95(3):254–7.
84. US Food and Drug Administration. Table of pharmacogenomic biomarkers in drug labeling. Available at: http://www.fda.gov/Drugs/ScienceResearch/Research Areas/Pharmacogenetics/ucm083378.htm. Accessed April 21, 2015.
85. Schwemm A, Brusig E, Anderegg S, et al. Environmental scan of pharmacogenomics coding: current practice and barriers. Pharmacy Health Information Technology Collaborative. 2015. Available at: http://www.pharmacyhit.org/ pdfs/workshop-documents/WG2-Post-2015-01.pdf. Accessed June 22, 2015.
86. O'Donnell PH, Danahey K, Jacobs M, et al. Adoption of a clinical pharmacogenomics implementation program during outpatient care: initial results of the University of Chicago "1,200 Patients Project". Am J Med Genet C Semin Med Genet 2014;166C(1):68–75.
87. Hoffman JM, Haidar CE, Wilkinson MR, et al. PG4KDS: a model for the clinical implementation of pre-emptive pharmacogenetics. Am J Med Genet C Semin Med Genet 2014;166C(1):45–55.
88. Pulley JM, Denny JC, Peterson JF, et al. Operational implementation of prospective genotyping for personalized medicine: the design of the Vanderbilt PREDICT project. Clin Pharmacol Ther 2012;92(1):87–95.
89. Weitzel KW, Elsey AR, Langaee TY, et al. Clinical pharmacogenetics implementation: approaches, successes, and challenges. Am J Med Genet C Semin Med Genet 2014;166C(1):56–67.
90. Owusu-Obeng A, Weitzel KW, Hatton RC, et al. Emerging roles for pharmacists in clinical implementation of pharmacogenomics. Pharmacotherapy 2014; 34(10):1102–12.
91. Johnson JA, Elsey AR, Clare-Salzler MJ, et al. Institutional profile: university of Florida and Shands hospital personalized medicine program: clinical implementation of pharmacogenetics. Pharmacogenomics 2013;14(7):723–6.
92. Shuldiner AR, Palmer K, Pakyz RE, et al. Implementation of pharmacogenetics: the university of Maryland personalized anti-platelet pharmacogenetics program. Am J Med Genet C Semin Med Genet 2014;166C(1):76–84.
93. Bielinski SJ, Olson JE, Pathak J, et al. Preemptive genotyping for personalized medicine: design of the right drug, right dose, right time-using genomic data to individualize treatment protocol. Mayo Clin Proc 2014;89(1):25–33.
94. Levy KD, Decker BS, Carpenter JS, et al. Prerequisites to implementing a pharmacogenomics program in a large health-care system. Clin Pharmacol Ther 2014;96(3):307–9.

95. Reiss SM. American Pharmacists Association. Integrating pharmacogenomics into pharmacy practice via medication therapy management. J Am Pharm Assoc (2003) 2011;51(6):e64–74.

96. Haga SB, Allen LaPointe NM, Moaddeb J, et al. Pilot study: incorporation of pharmacogenetic testing in medication therapy management services. Pharmacogenomics 2014;15(14):1729–37.

97. Swen JJ, van der Straaten T, Wessels JA, et al. Feasibility of pharmacy-initiated pharmacogenetic screening for CYP2D6 and CYP2C19. Eur J Clin Pharmacol 2012;68(4):363–70.

98. Moaddeb J, Mills R, Haga SB. Community pharmacists' experience with pharmacogenetic testing. J Am Pharm Assoc (2003) 2015;55(6):587–94.

99. Crews KR, Cross SJ, McCormick JN, et al. Development and implementation of a pharmacist-managed clinical pharmacogenetics service. Am J Health Syst Pharm 2011;68(2):143–50.

100. Haga SB, LaPointe NM, Cho A, et al. Pilot study of pharmacist-assisted delivery of pharmacogenetic testing in a primary care setting. Pharmacogenomics 2014; 15(13):1677–86.

101. Haga SB, Moaddeb J, Mills R, et al. Incorporation of pharmacogenetic testing into medication therapy management. Pharmacogenomics 2015;16(17): 1931–41.

102. O'Connor SK, Ferreri SP, Michaels NM, et al. Exploratory planning and implementation of a pilot pharmacogenetic program in a community pharmacy. Pharmacogenomics 2012;13(8):955–62.

103. Haga SB, Allen LaPointe NM, Moaddeb J. Challenges to integrating pharmacogenetic testing into medication therapy management. J Manag Care Spec Pharm 2015;21(4):346–52.

104. Delafuente JC. Pharmacokinetic and pharmacodynamic alterations in the geriatric patient. Consult Pharm 2008;23(4):324–34.

105. Bressler R, Bahl JJ. Principles of drug therapy for the elderly patient. Mayo Clin Proc 2003;78(12):1564–77.

106. Relling MV, Klein TE. CPIC: clinical pharmacogenetics implementation consortium of the pharmacogenomics research network. Clin Pharmacol Ther 2011;89(3):464–7.

107. Alexander KM, Divine HS, Hanna CR, et al. Implementation of personalized medicine services in community pharmacies: perceptions of independent community pharmacists. J Am Pharm Assoc (2003) 2014;54(5):510–7.

108. Haga SB, O'Daniel JM, Tindall GM, et al. Survey of US public attitudes toward pharmacogenetic testing. Pharmacogenomics J 2012;12(3):197–204.

109. Latif DA, McKay AB. Pharmacogenetics and pharmacogenomics instruction in colleges and schools of pharmacy in the United States. Am J Pharm Educ 2005;69(2):152–6.

110. Johansen Taber KA, Dickinson BD. Pharmacogenomic knowledge gaps and educational resource needs among physicians in selected specialties. Pharmgenomics Pers Med 2014;7:145–62.

111. Suther S, Goodson P. Barriers to the provision of genetic services by primary care physicians: a systematic review of the literature. Genet Med 2003;5(2): 70–6.

112. Mikat-Stevens NA, Larson IA, Tarini BA. Primary-care providers' perceived barriers to integration of genetics services: a systematic review of the literature. Genet Med 2015;17(3):169–76.

113. Peterson JF, Field JR, Shi Y, et al. Attitudes of clinicians following large-scale pharmacogenomics implementation. Pharmacogenomics J 2015;16(4):393–8.

114. Haga SB, Tindall G, O'Daniel JM. Professional perspectives about pharmacogenetic testing and managing ancillary findings. Genet Test Mol Biomarkers 2012; 16(1):21–4.

115. Ferro WG, Kuo GM, Jenkins JF, et al. Pharmacist education in the era of genomic medicine. J Am Pharm Assoc (2003) 2012;52(5):e113–21.

116. McCullough KB, Formea CM, Berg KD, et al. Assessment of the pharmacogenomics educational needs of pharmacists. Am J Pharm Educ 2011;75(3):51.

117. de Denus S, Letarte N, Hurlimann T, et al. An evaluation of pharmacists' expectations towards pharmacogenomics. Pharmacogenomics 2013;14(2):165–75.

118. Gottesman O, Kuivaniemi H, Tromp G, et al. The electronic medical records and genomics (eMERGE) network: past, present, and future. Genet Med 2013; 15(10):761–71.

119. Haga SB, Tindall G, O'Daniel JM. Public perspectives about pharmacogenetic testing and managing ancillary findings. Genet Test Mol Biomarkers 2012;16(3): 193–7.

120. Houwink EJ, van Luijk SJ, Henneman L, et al. Genetic educational needs and the role of genetics in primary care: a focus group study with multiple perspectives. BMC Fam Pract 2011;12:5.

121. Haga SB, O'Daniel JM, Tindall GM, et al. Public attitudes toward ancillary information revealed by pharmacogenetic testing under limited information conditions. Genet Med 2011;13(8):723–8.

122. Cogent Research C. Americans skeptical of physicians' knowledge of genomics. Business Wire. 2011. Available at: http://www.businesswire.com/news/home/20110125006349/en/Americans-Skeptical-Physicians%E2%80%99-Knowledge-Genomics. Accessed March 23, 2016.

123. Kirk M, Calzone K, Arimori N, et al. Genetics-genomics competencies and nursing regulation. J Nurs Scholarsh 2011;43(2):107–16.

124. Murphy JE, Green JS, Adams LA, et al. Pharmacogenomics in the curricula of colleges and schools of pharmacy in the United States. Am J Pharm Educ 2010;74(1):7.

125. American Society of Health-System Pharmacists. ASHP statement on the pharmacist's role in clinical Pharmacogenomics. Am J Health Syst Pharm 2015; 72(7):579–81.

126. Johnson SG. Leading clinical pharmacogenomics implementation: advancing pharmacy practice. Am J Health Syst Pharm 2015;72(15):1324–8.

127. Michaels NM, Jenkins GF, Pruss DL, et al. Retrospective analysis of community pharmacists' recommendations in the North Carolina Medicaid medication therapy management program. J Am Pharm Assoc (2003) 2010;50(3):347–53.

128. DeName B, Divine H, Nicholas A, et al. Identification of medication-related problems and health care provider acceptance of pharmacist recommendations in the DiabetesCARE program. J Am Pharm Assoc (2003) 2008;48(6):731–6.

129. Doucette WR, McDonough RP, Klepser D, et al. Comprehensive medication therapy management: identifying and resolving drug-related issues in a community pharmacy. Clin Ther 2005;27(7):1104–11.

130. Perera PN, Guy MC, Sweaney AM, et al. Evaluation of prescriber responses to pharmacist recommendations communicated by fax in a medication therapy management program (MTMP). J Manag Care Pharm 2011;17(5):345–54.

Geriatric Polypharmacy
Two Physicians' Personal Perspectives

Zhe Chen, MD*, Anthony Buonanno, MD, MBA

KEYWORDS

- Polypharmacy • Potentially inappropriate medications • Deprescribing

KEY POINTS

- There are many studies showing potentially inappropriate medications (PIMs) being prescribed in the geriatric population.
- People with the greatest burden of PIM and polypharmacy are generally 80 years and older, due to multiple comorbidities and lower life expectancy; PIMs prescribed to older people are highly prevalent in the United States and Europe, 12% in the outpatient population and 40% in nursing home residents.
- In today's environment of Press Ganey surveys and Hospital Consumer Assessment of Healthcare Providers and Systems, physicians may be pressured into prescribing unnecessary or nonindicated drugs.
- Deprescribing is defined as the systematic process of identifying and discontinuing drugs in instances in which potential harms outweigh potential benefits within the context of an individual's care goals, current level of functioning, life expectancy, values, and preferences.
- Health care over the past century has innovated tremendously in biomedical science and pharmaceutical development.

Being a clinical provider in today's health care environment has become complex with more levels of care to negotiate. Additionally, there are more types of medical practitioners involved in patient care. Information is compiled and updated frantically, and being a physician is like drinking water from a fire hydrant. Efficiency is replacing the intimate patient-physician relationship because of skyrocketing costs in a 3-party system. A system previously guided by a physician's thought process has become complex with multiple drivers and competing agendas. Who is caught in the middle of this complexity? Senior citizens. As we evolve into the new quality model, new problems and complexities occur. Numerous protocols and guidelines necessitate the initiation of drugs for given diagnoses and aggressive treatments. This article discusses

LVPG Hospital Medicine at Cedar Crest, 1200 S. Cedar Crest Boulevard, 3rd Floor Anderson Wing, Allentown, PA 18103, USA
* Corresponding author.
E-mail address: Zhe.Chen@lvhn.org

Clin Geriatr Med 33 (2017) 283–288
http://dx.doi.org/10.1016/j.cger.2017.01.008
0749-0690/17/© 2017 Elsevier Inc. All rights reserved.

geriatric.theclinics.com

geriatric polypharmacy from 2 practitioners' viewpoints: Zhe Chen, MD, discusses the point of view of a physician provider, and Anthony Buonanno, MD, discusses the provider's role in his or her own family.

DR CHEN

Remembering the first time I felt the problem as an intern, I was admitting a 72-year-old paraplegic man. As I was placing orders, I examined the home medication list and was astonished. I turned through 3 to 4 pages. It was the largest medication list I had ever seen. Not knowing where to start, I could not help but stare. Finally, I conjured the will to enter his home medications one by one. Moving down the list, the interaction warning screen started popping up more. Toward the end, my senior medical resident was calling, "we still have more patients to admit." I was clicking the override button without much thought. If another doctor prescribed it, he or she must have thought it through. Since that start of my education, I have grown used to these long lists.

Remembering another moment, I was a resident and the patient was an elderly man. He was very tall, with a large scar on his arm. He always answered my questions in the most honest tone of voice. He had a history of unexplained syncope, blacking out episodes for which he saw many doctors. He saw a cardiologist and wore a long-term cardiac monitor that ruled out an abnormal heart rhythm. He also had a continuous electroencephalogram that proved these were not seizures. I asked him why he was still on the Levetiracetam 1000 mg twice daily. He just shrugged his shoulders and said "I don't know," not remembering when he started it, or why he was still taking it. All his previous testing had been done at another hospital. I brought this to the attention of my attending, wanting to taper it down and stop it. However, there was reluctance in her voice: "I am not a neurologist. Call and try to speak with the person who prescribed it." So I called the outside hospital, gave the patient's name and date of birth, and tried to find the neurologist. Ultimately, I found out this doctor had already moved to another hospital. After an entire hour into our visit, I went back to my attending expressing my frustration. I told her I was confident these events were not seizures based on his story. Besides, he was still having these episodes regardless of the medication. She reluctantly agreed to decrease the dose, but requested I make a referral to another neurologist. This is another hidden cost created by polypharmacy.

As I reflect on my education and what I was taught about polypharmacy, I vaguely remember the lectures: mentioning the problem, the Beers and Screening Tool of Older Persons' Prescriptions (STOPP) criteria, and the challenges ahead. Having been taught the concepts and introduced to the problem, did I really know how to face it directly? I have never encountered a prompt in the electronic medical record stating "this medication meets the Beers criteria as a potentially inappropriate medication, please consider addressing it." I do not remember an attending telling me to spend dedicated time reviewing the patient's medications, seeing if any of them are appropriate for his or her age. Physicians are expected to finish a visit with a patient in 15 to 20 minutes. Many insurance policies limit the number of doctor appointments each year. Can I reasonably schedule a patient to solely discuss cutting back medications? Such a visit would require contacting certain subspecialists in a timely manner. Our health care system, with patient care fractured into multiple providers, is not designed to address an issue that requires this type of integrated approach.

There are many studies showing potentially inappropriate medications (PIMs) being prescribed in the geriatric population. People with the greatest burden of PIM and polypharmacy are generally 80 years and older, due to multiple comorbidities and lower life expectancy. PIMs prescribed to older people are highly prevalent in the United States and Europe, 12% in the outpatient population and 40% in nursing home residents.[1] The Beers criteria was one of the first tools described in 1991, which was simply 30 drugs to be avoided in the elderly. These criteria have been updated numerous times. Other tools, such as Screening Tool to Alert doctors to Right Treatment (START) and STOPP, also have been developed. However, we have not found a place in our health care system to formally apply these tools. They exist in the vacuum of academic literature, discussed at conferences, but not truly imbedded into habitual practice of most physicians.

Patient expectations also drive polypharmacy. With an increasing focus on the provider to take action to increase patient satisfaction, prescribing is seen by patients as a sign of caring. Another one of my patients was an 89-year-old woman with dementia who had not been eating well for the past few weeks. Her blood pressure was low. She improved with intravenous fluids, and when her urinalysis showed a positive leukocyte esterase, and positive bacteria, the emergency room team started antibiotics. She did not complain of urinary symptoms. She had no fevers and no elevation in her white blood cell count. I was not confident she had a true urinary tract infection. Thus, I discussed with the patient's husband the possibility of stopping the antibiotic and observing her. As soon as I mentioned stopping antibiotics, I saw his nervous glances. "I feel very uncomfortable with that idea," he said. Some time had passed, and then I was called back into the room. Her husband had requested another doctor to see the patient. "I just don't want you to not give her any antibiotics." I proceeded to sit down and talk to him in detail about the reasons why I felt stopping antibiotics was the most appropriate course of action. I explained the increasing problem of antibiotic resistance, and the problem with using only a urine test to make the diagnosis without clear symptoms. I inquired more deeply about her dementia, and learned about her decline over the past few months. Her husband started crying, and I sat with him for a little more than an hour. We proceeded to discuss her goals of care.

There are few studies on patient satisfaction and expectations with regard to prescriptions and ordering medications. In one study in the *British Medical Journal* in 1997, patient hopes for prescriptions exceeded both doctors' perception of these hopes and their level of prescribing.[2] Even though prescriptions were written less often than patients hoped, the writing of nonindicated prescriptions was primarily associated with the doctors' sense of feeling pressured. A third of prescriptions written were either not indicated or hoped for, 3% being neither indicated nor hoped for.[2] This tells us that in today's environment of Press Ganey surveys and Hospital Consumer Assessment of Healthcare Providers and Systems, physicians may be pressured into prescribing unnecessary or nonindicated drugs. Often, if there is sufficient time, a physician can counsel the patient as to why a medication is not indicated in a particular case. However, this counseling often requires the development of trust, and the patient having a sense that the physician understands what he or she feels. The physician must listen and explain, and the patient must believe that the physician has the patient's best interest in mind. Regardless of what the doctor says, if there is not enough time spent during the encounter, that relationship and trust cannot develop. There is time taken away during a visit because of a variety of screenings that must take place during a patient assessment, such as asking questions about falls, depression, and abuse. This is impossible to achieve in our health care system, which demands high efficiency and throughput. The next patient to be seen is invariably waiting in a clinician's cue of work.

DR BUONANNO

Geriatric polypharmacy has affected my father, who never liked to take medications from as far back as I can remember as a little boy through his old age. He is a pharmacist who has always felt people took too many medications. As a son of a pharmacist, who graduated pharmacy school and practiced, one would think my family is protected. I entered medical school as a pharmacist, and became board-certified in internal medicine. My father owned a small drugstore in Brooklyn, NY, and he practiced in a way that made me proud to be his son. He never understood the third-party payment system. I remember him telling me, it will never work. People come in for a prescription and you give them something that somebody else pays for. They do not understand they are paying through salary reduction and insurance premiums. Because it was prepaid, people want their money's worth. Well, he was right no doubt. He worked hard his entire life, and was able to sell his store for pennies on the dollar after the big chain stores moved into the area. He was in his sixties. He became an employee at a mail-order pharmacy company. He needed to work for the health insurance coverage.

While in my residency, he telephoned me asking when I was coming home for a visit. He told me he was having chest pain, "so you should bring your stethoscope." I told him to go to the doctor's immediately, but he refused. My brother put him on a plane to meet me, and we went to the cardiologist's office. He took out a bottle of nitroglycerine and showed my colleague the bottle, telling him the chest pain started 12 years ago, but now 4 or 5 doses does not take away the pain. Within a week, he had a 5-vessel coronary artery bypass graft. Again, he is an intelligent pharmacist, avoiding care. On discharge, he had a whole new regimen of medications. He worked at a mail-order pharmacy, but with his coverage, he still could not afford the drug copays. He next went to the Department of Veterans Affairs (VA) to get his prescriptions at a much lower cost. The VA uses a formulary system, so his medications were changed. He went from no drugs to 7 in a blink of an eye (metoprolol, lisinopril, amlodipine, furosemide, simvastatin, aspirin, and clopidogrel). Not feeling well, he did what many seniors do, experimenting with starting and stopping medications. He would start his blood pressure meds 2 to 3 days before a doctor's visit, so as not to anger his physician. He also wanted to avoid having more medication prescribed for him. His blood pressure was still not controlled, so they added hydralazine.

Months after being encouraged to take his medication, he was aging quickly. He started to work at a local retail chain pharmacy, and had a syncopal episode at work. He refused to go with the ambulance, and his store manager called me while emergency medical services was with him. They did not take him to the hospital, because his son, the doctor, could come and get him. I took him to where I worked. He was washed out, pale and short of breath. After his initial workup, he was found to have a hemoglobin of 8, chest radiograph with pulmonary edema, and a creatinine of 3. I was confused as to why this was happening. However, after listening to him tell his story, I realized I was unaware of how much pain he truly was in. He told the admitting physician he was using nonsteroidal anti-inflammatory drugs (NSAIDs) multiple times a day for many days. His range of motion was very limited, and he was losing mobility. Also, evaluation revealed a positive antihistone antibody during his inpatient stay. In summary, after being on hydralazine for a year, he developed drug-induced lupus erythematosus, causing myalgia, which led him to take NSAIDs that caused renal insufficiency, contributing to congestive heart failure and a gastric ulcer and subsequent anemia, all leading to syncope. After stopping the hydralazine, he was doing much better within 3 to 4 months.

Years went by, and my dad continued to work until the age of 80 years. He subsequently developed rheumatoid arthritis. He became more and more immobile and was living in his own condo near me. With support from family and a homecare agency 4 hours a day, he remained independent. More medications had been added: a methotrexate trial, prednisone, proton pump inhibiter, hydroxychloroquine, and around-the-clock acetaminophen. It was obvious he was not doing well against father time. The nearly fatal blow was an episode of herpes zoster leading to tremendous pain. He was placed on lidocaine ointment, gabapentin, and tramadol. He became incoherent; one will never know whether it was the pain or the medications. It probably was a combination of everything. He was now on 13 or 14 medications and he was falling more than 3 to 4 times a week. He was impulsive and confused. I was frustrated because no matter what I tried, it made him worse. My siblings were frustrated as well. I felt I was letting the family down, and more importantly my dad. I took him to rheumatologists, gastroenterologists, and cardiologists and had him see the best internist in town. He went in and out of the hospital and short-term rehabilitation facilities too numerous to count. Although my doctor card made it easy to navigate the system, in some respects it hurt him.

As physicians, we want to help people and have the best intentions. When someone is in pain, what are our tools? A medication, physical therapy, and surgery are bridges but not cures. He eventually took more pain medications and stopped eating and drinking. I called my family members and we discussed hospice. I remember sitting outside a pizzeria, thinking he loves pizza and has not had it for a long time. I bought a pie, and brought it to his house. I decided to stop all but his pain medications as he became obtunded. The next day he woke up some more, I heated up the pizza and he had a big smile on his face. He asked me where the Coke was. He started eating and drinking and woke up, making sense again. I wish the story ended with he lived happily ever after. He is alive and now bedbound and he is on minimal medications. He eventually went into a long-term care facility. I am not blaming medication for this story, but it was a big part of his history. My colleagues were great, and did all the right things. But sometimes we just need a slice and a Coke.

It is easy to realize the problem and give it a term, polypharmacy. But what is the solution? Is it ethical to try to cut costs on the system by targeting senior citizens' prescriptions? Should we attack the medications or prevent the adverse events? More comorbidities and medication use correlate strongly with nursing home placement, impaired mobility, morbidity, hospitalizations, and death.[3] The next generation of guidelines is being developed for deprescribing medications. Deprescribing is defined as the systematic process of identifying and discontinuing drugs in instances in which potential harms outweigh potential benefits within the context of an individual's care goals, current level of functioning, life expectancy, values, and preferences.[4] This part of the care continuum (is the medication truly worth taking) needs continued assessment. Physicians often fail to include the duration and potential adverse effects when prescribing. In a study published in the Archives of Internal Medicine,[5] 44 physicians were evaluated on prescribing medication to 185 patients. They were graded on a 5-point medication index (name, purpose, directions, duration, and potential adverse effects) with an average of 3.1 of the 5 elements being addressed by clinicians. The duration of therapy and adverse events were explained only 34% and 35% of the time. The investigator felt that poor communication may be due to lack of time with a patient, and overreliance on pharmacists educating patients.[5] Yet, many factors affect the pharmacist-patient interaction. Pharmacies allow patients to sign a waiver for pharmacist counseling, and many patients are using mail-order pharmacies as well. Pharmacists are feeling the same pressure as physicians with regard to work volume and staffing.

However, we believe there is hope. Health care constantly changes. Many networks are using pharmacists in unique ways to provide recommendations about evaluating and deprescribing medications. Affordable Care Organizations are trialing interdisciplinary teams to address neglected areas of service and organization, and to avoid overlap. Health care over the past century has innovated tremendously in biomedical science, and pharmaceutical development. In this century, innovation will arise in health care organization and infrastructure, and with enough courage and determination, develop a system to tackle this problem.

REFERENCES

1. Gallagher P, Barry P, O'Mahony D. Inappropriate prescribing in the elderly. J Clin Pharm Ther 2007;32:113–21.
2. The influence of patients' hopes of receiving a prescription on doctors' perceptions and the decision to prescribe: a questionnaire survey. Available at: http://www.bmj.com/content/315/7121/1506.full.print. Accessed May 9, 2016.
3. Garfinkel D, Mangin D. Feasibility study of a systematic approach for discontinuation of multiple medications in older adults addressing polypharmacy. Arch Intern Med 2010;170(18):1648–54.
4. Scott I, Hilmer S, Reeve E, et al. Reducing inappropriate polypharmacy: the process of deprescribing. JAMA Intern Med 2015;175(5):827–34.
5. Tarn DM, Heritage J, Paterniti DA, et al. Physician communication when prescribing new medications. Arch Intern Med 2006;166(17):1855–62.

Index

Note Page numbers of article titles are in **boldface** type.

A

Adverse drug events, and polypharmacy, in critically ill older adults, factors associated with, 197
Affordable Care Act, 245
American Geriatrics Society Beers Criteria, 226, 248
    polypharmacy reduction strategies and, 180–181
Antimicrobial stewardship, 250–251
Antipsychotics, or dexmedetomidine, in treatment of, evaluation of, 195, 196

C

Centers for Disease Control and Prevention, overuse of antibiotics and, 250
Centers for Medicare and Medicaid Services, financial incentives for part D sponsors, 160
    medication therapy management, star measure rating, 158–159
        support for, **153–164**
Critically ill older adults, polypharmacy and adverse drug events in, factors associated with, 197
    polypharmacy and delirium in, **189–203**

D

Delirium, antipsychotic or dexmedetomidine treatment of, evaluation of, 195, 196
    in critically ill older adults, 191–192
    in intensive care unit, risk factors for and causes of, 198
    intensive care unit medications associated with, 193
    medication-related, strategies to reduce, 198
    nonmedication risk factors for, 192
    polypharmacy and, in critically ill older adults, **189–203**
    polypharmacy as risk factor for, 192–194
    treatment of, polypharmacy as sequelae of, 195, 196
Dementia, and behavioral and psychological symptoms of dementia, 249–250
Deprescribing, barriers and pitfalls to, 171–172
    definition of, 166–167, 209, 241–242
    patient preferences in, 167–171
    preferences in, role of patient in, **165–175**
    process of, 167, 168
Dexmedetomidine, or antipsychotics, in treatment of delirium, evaluation of, 195, 196
Diabetes management, 251
Drug reactions, adverse, as cause of death, 226

E

Electronic health records, impact on patient safety, 231

Clin Geriatr Med 33 (2017) 289–292
http://dx.doi.org/10.1016/S0749-0690(17)30028-9
0749-0690/17

geriatric.theclinics.com

Moving?

Make sure your subscription moves with you!

To notify us of your new address, find your **Clinics Account Number** (located on your mailing label above your name), and contact customer service at:

Email: journalscustomerservice-usa@elsevier.com

800-654-2452 (subscribers in the U.S. & Canada)
314-447-8871 (subscribers outside of the U.S. & Canada)

Fax number: 314-447-8029

Elsevier Health Sciences Division
Subscription Customer Service
3251 Riverport Lane
Maryland Heights, MO 63043

*To ensure uninterrupted delivery of your subscription, please notify us at least 4 weeks in advance of move.

Printed and bound by CPI Group (UK) Ltd, Croydon, CR0 4YY

07/10/2024

01040502-0015